Running for My Life, Winning for CMT

Memoirs of an Athlete
with Charcot-Marie-Tooth

Running for My Life, Winning for CMT

Memoirs of an Athlete
with Charcot-Marie-Tooth

Christine Wodke

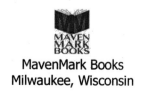

MavenMark Books
Milwaukee, Wisconsin

Published by
MavenMark Books
An imprint of HenschelHAUS Publishing, Inc.
2625 S. Greeley St. Suite 201
Milwaukee, WI 53207
www. henschelHAUSbooks.com

All HenschelHAUS titles, imprints, and distributed lines
are available at special quantity discounts for educational,
institutional, fund-raising, or sales promotion.

ISBN: 978159598-282-7
E-ISBN: 978159598-283-4
LCCN: 20139523000

Printed in the United States of America.

A portion of the proceeds from the sale of this book go to fund
research and raise awareness for Charcot-Marie-Tooth (CMT).

I run because I can, when I get tired I remember those who can't run, what they would give to have this simple gift I take for grated and I run harder for them, I know they would do the same for me.
—Unknown

This book is dedicated to the members of Team CMT, especially those affected with CMT. Thank you for your courage and determination to be athletes in spite of the challenges you face. You inspire me. Thank you to those on the team who joined to support affected friends and family members. Your love and support mean more than you will ever know.

This book is also for the 155,000 Americans and 2.6 million people worldwide affected by CMT. This book was written to give you a voice and to put a face to CMT.

Team CMT members, walk, swim, run, and cycle for those who can't to raise awareness and to funds for research to find treatments and a cure.

Thank you to our partner, the Hereditary Neuropathy Foundation. In HNF President Allison Moore, we found a supporter, friend, and fellow athlete. I am forever grateful to the HNF and our team members for their support and commitment to our mission to raise awareness of Charcot-Marie-Tooth and to educate the public on the challenges those affected by CMT face.

Table of Contents

Foreword

I am delighted that Chris Wodke published her memoir of how one's perseverance and dedication can change the world. Chris tells her story of determination that goes beyond the limits while living with a common, inherited neuromuscular disease, Charcot-Marie-Tooth (CMT), a progressive, debilitating condition for which there is currently no cure.

Chris is an inspiration as she overcomes obstacles of training with CMT, such as exhaustion and injury, while working a full-time job and managing Team CMT, a group of athletes who share in our mission to raise awareness for CMT and funds for research.

CMT is a disease that can remain hidden for some. It can separate and divide, from early days of a child with CMT falling behind in gym class, to a teen unable to wear high heels to homecoming or making the football team, to adults who struggle with small tasks around the house or office. CMT can feel like it's just you, alone, against the world.

Chris's physical and emotional journey puts this disease where it should be, in the spotlight, and focuses us all on the positive things one can do to embrace and live life to the fullest with CMT. By merging her platform of Team CMT with the Hereditary Neuropathy Foundation's dedication to raising awareness, we create a strong and vocal community that will one day find a cure for this disease.

This is a passionate story of how one young woman, elite athlete and my friend, has changed the world and helped so many. Chris's experiences will resonate with the millions around the world who are affected by CMT, as well as anyone who sets a goal up high and then clamors to reach it.

Allison Moore
CEO and Founder
Consumer Advisor Associate
Hereditary Neuropathy Foundation

Chapter 1
Running for My Life

The miracle isn't that I finished.
The miracle is that I had the courage to start.
—John Bingham, American marathon runner and author

I have several vivid memories from childhood. I spent most of my grade school life with perpetually skinned knees because I was always falling. I was a clumsy kid and I was slow. I grew up in Milwaukee as one of seven kids. I was right in the middle, three boys older and two boys and a girl younger. Being a quiet middle child, it was easy to be overlooked and I learned the art of blending in early in life.

Milwaukee is an ethnic city, mostly German and Polish. My family was German Lutheran so of course, I was sent to Bethany Lutheran grade school. Germans are very orderly and rule-oriented. Our teachers loved us but also managed us with strict discipline. One of the most vivid memories I have of grade school is when the entire school of 200 students walked the six blocks from our school building to the church that sponsored our school. We did it for church service at the start and end of school year and when we practiced for Christmas service. I remember walking two by two through the neighborhood in one very quiet and orderly line. Acting out brought corporal punishment and there was very little misbehavior.

There was no school violence, truancy, or backtalk to teachers. It really was a different time.

I also remember running relay races outside on the playground. We were split into groups of five or six kids. We lined up and when the whistle blew, we ran to some point, turned around and ran back, tagged the next person on our team and repeated. The first team to get all the kids back and forth won. I was always being yelled at for being slow. Everyone likes to win and I was not an asset to any team I was on. I can still hear one of my classmates screaming at me. "You are so slow!"

Slow and clumsy also made a bad combination for the grade-school game we played called "Run for Your Life." I think it was the particular invention of one of our teachers, whom I both loved and feared. I liked him so much. We were the lucky class that had him assigned 4th, 6th, and 7th grade. My favorite teacher and I sparred many times in our years together. I was a straight A student except for handwriting and gym. At my school, neat handwriting mattered. Once, in front of the whole class, he asked how I expected to write a letter to my boyfriend with such messy handwriting. I looked him straight in the eye and said I'd type. I never was one to back off from a fight, even with a teacher. I never got bullied in school and that might be why.

In my kid memories, my "favorite" teacher was huge. Red hair, red beard, and a big stocky guy who look like he had played football in college. He had a yardstick wrapped in blue tape he used to wield discipline. He once cracked that stick on his glass desktop and shattered it. He thought nothing about grabbing a kid out of a line, lifting him off the ground, putting him at eye level, and loudly asking "What are you doing?" That was the 1960s and we attended a private school. Not the kind of wimpy education kids get today. I swear kids today go through life wrapped in bubble wrap.

The ultimate contest of wills took place during "Run for Your Life." It went like this. The massive Mr. O would stand at center court of our gym basketball court. In his massive hands, he held a red rubber playground ball. The four corners of the gym were "safe" zones. The whole class started at one corner, the gym entrance. When he blew his whistle, you were fair game. You had to run to the next safe zone. As you ran past, he would try and pick you off with one of the many red rubber playground balls he had in his procession. When you were hit, you were out. He seemed to take sadistic pleasure in picking us off one by one. The last one standing won.

We were like gazelles being hunted. He was the predator and we were the prey. The weak and the slow were picked off first. When the rubber ball hit you, it stung and left a mark. I think I still have marks and even today, can feel the terror of the whistle blowing. The strategy was to try and be in the crowd for protection. It is amazing I ever ran a step after being subjected to "Run for Your life." I think the game has now been banned except to torture terrorists. I was never, ever the last one standing.

I had to play "Run for Your Life" many times during grade school. Not only was Mr. O my grade-level teacher, he was also the gym teacher. I had gym at least three times a week. I never knew when "Run for Your Life" or some similar torture was on the agenda. It's no wonder that when I had a choice in high school, I dropped gym. It is a miracle I ever ran again.

On the other hand, I loved being active outside of gym class. My brothers and I rode our bikes, swam, played football, tag, and baseball. We watched lots of TV like any kid in the 60s, but we also played outside a lot. No soccer leagues, no play dates, no moms hovering nearby. It was just good old running around the neighborhood with my brothers and our friends. No one blew a whistle, trying to pick me off or measuring how fast I ran. It was just play and it was fun. I have continued to be active my whole life because of those enjoyable moments.

My school gym was also the source of my greatest sports moment. We played whiffle ball—plastic ball, plastic bat, and set up inside the same gym. I was no better at whiffle ball than anything else athletic. Mr. O always pitched. He could throw a mean fastball and it stung if you got in the way. But one day, I hit a home run off of Mr. O. Yup, hit the corner doors, which meant an automatic home run. I got to touch 'em all. Even better was seeing the stunned look on Mr. O's face as I headed around the bases. No single sports moment in my life has ever been sweeter knowing how I had bested him.

So sometimes life is like that. Sometimes you feel like you're running for your life. Sometimes you feel the sting of getting hit. Other times, you're rounding third and heading for home. You just have to stay in there and keep swinging. You never know when you will connect for that big hit.

Today, many games are now banned in schools because they promote competition and hurt self-esteem. Being the slowest in the class didn't damage me. I found ways to excel that didn't involve relay races and running for my life. I learned to work really hard to overcome any limitations. I've found that hard work can be just as important as talent.

Competition made me strong and gave me a keen work ethic. I have Mr. O to thank for that perseverance and ability to keep on going despite the odds.

Remember the screaming kid from the relay race? I still hear his voice inside my head and use it to motivate me when I run. I bet he is sitting on a sofa somewhere with a beer in one hand and a remote in the other. He would have to catch me now to yell at me.

I chose not to let the experience crush me; I've used it to motivate me. Sometimes I still feel like that slow kid cowering in the corner. But when the whistle blows, I run.

See if you can keep up.

Chapter 2
The Day that Changed My Life

When one door of happiness closes, another opens, but often we look so long at the closed door, that we do not see the one that has been opened up for us.
—Helen Keller

Sometimes we have days that change the course of our life. That day happened to me on a Father's Day 1999 and I can't even remember most of it. I'd planned a family brunch with my dad and brothers, but other events got in the way.

My life had been pretty uneventful up to that point. I was still living in Milwaukee and working for the local electric utility as a technical trainer. I had earned two engineering degrees from the University of Wisconsin–Milwaukee. I held a variety of jobs in the field, including research engineer on defense projects, a production manager assembling circuit boards, and a product safety engineer. I had survived two job layoffs and had been in my current job for six months.

I was single and the proud owner of a vintage duplex I had restored on the south side of Milwaukee in the Bay View neighborhood. When Milwaukee was planned, the city founders designed a park into every neighborhood. My own neighborhood park was right across the street. My home office boasted a lovely view of the park's lily pond.

I love Bay View because it is ethnically and economically diverse. It once was the site of the largest steel rolling mill in the world. Local mill workers came from Wales and England and were joined later by immigrants from Italy and Poland. The neighborhood still reflects those roots. You can still see the cottages from the mill workers and the mill superintendent home. Bay View was annexed into the city of Milwaukee in 1894, but has always retained a strong and separate community feel.

After college, I had lived on the east side of Milwaukee. Very trendy, but very transient. Bay View and Milwaukee are the kind of places where people grow up, go to school, get a job, raise and their families. Kids grow up in Bay View and stay to raise their families. I just loved the stable and family feeling of the neighborhood. My neighbors had lived in their house for over 30 years.

I was a transplant who had grown up on the west side of Milwaukee in a largely German-speaking neighborhood. By the time I grew up, the neighborhood of my childhood had changed to a high crime area, riddled with drug houses and vacant lots. Staying was not an option.

That Father's Day was a gorgeous warm June Sunday and I got up and went for a bike ride early that morning. Despite my shaky athletic start in grade school, I was now one of many runners who lined up for local running races on weekends. I started running in college with one of my engineering school friends to get in shape for downhill skiing.

After college, my roommate Cheryl Monnat invited me and her fiancé to join them at a local race. I was slow but I was hooked. I entered lots of local races and had fun even though I was not fast.

Years of races later, I dated a local running coach for a bit. After we stopped dating, I hired him to coach me since he counted many top athletes as his clients. He taught me how to do speed work, tempo runs, and all the other things I needed to become faster. It worked.

I became a threat to place in the top three in my age group in smaller races. Biking was part of my cross-training and that Sunday, I was training for the Lake Front Marathon in Milwaukee in October. When training for my first marathon, I had discovered that my body could not handle running every day. So I alternated biking with running. This marathon would be my fifth.

I remember getting out of bed that morning. The next thing I remember was coming out of a CAT scanner in St. Luke's ER in Milwaukee at 2 o'clock that afternoon.

Apparently a car had opened its door into my path as I biked up the street right outside Immaculate Conception church. It figures that I would get hit outside a church, since I was skipping church to do my bike ride. I hit the car door so hard that the bike helmet I was wearing left ridges in my head. I didn't know it at the time, but I had a head injury and a broken collar bone. I don't remember any of it. According to an EMT on the scene, I kept repeating myself, a classic sign of head injury.

I have a vague recollection of being strapped to a backboard and lifted into an ambulance. I know from taking care of patients as a member of the National Ski Patrol that people are only strapped to a backboard if there is the likelihood of a head or spine injury. A spine injury means paralysis.

I wiggled my toes, so I knew I wasn't paralyzed. I remember fading out as the ambulance started moving.

What I didn't know at the time was that I would never be the same as an athlete. I had been a 7:30-minute-mile runner prior to the accident. My fastest mile was 6:54 minutes. Not considered an elite athlete's speed, but still pretty good for an amateur athlete.

I would usually pick up an age group award at local runs. After the accident, my mile-per-minute time was two minutes or more slower. It would be some time before I knew why. But on that day, athletic performance was the last thing on my mind.

The ER doctor came to talk to me after my CAT scan. He asked me if I remembered talking to him. I didn't, even though he had spoken to me twice before the scan. I was admitted for observation and spent the next two days getting tests. To this day, I still don't remember anything else that happened. I was lucky I had worn a helmet; a biker not wearing a helmet was killed in a similar accident in the Milwaukee area later that week.

Because of the memory loss, the docs brought some of my family in. Two of my brothers arrived. I kept telling everyone I had an important meeting at work the next day and they couldn't keep me in the hospital. One of my brother's later told me I was so out of it that I kept asking when we were going to brunch with Dad.

I was assigned a neurologist in the hospital because there was concern there may have been an underlying condition causing my memory loss. I remember every time I saw him, he tested my memory. He'd name the same three objects—a ball, a flag and a Christmas tree—and ask me to repeat them back. For crying out loud, the objects never changed. Who wouldn't remember them? I couldn't make change for a dollar or remember anything else for months—but I could remember those three objects. They're still firmly planted in my memory over a decade later.

The neurologist decided to test my reflexes and found they were much diminished. That was not news to me, because I had always had sketchy knee reflexes. He then did nerve conduction tests and found my nerve conduction was very slow. He tested me for all kinds of conditions like multiple sclerosis (MS) and amyotrophic lateral sclerosis (ALS). I drew the line at a spinal tap. All the tests came back negative. He was scaring the crap out of me.

A friend of mine asked if I had some disease that began in middle age, would I really want to know right then? I said no and never went back to the doctor.

For months after the accident, I struggled with classic head-injury symptoms: vertigo, memory loss, mood swings, and lack of tolerance for noise. The doctors never gave me any recommendations about what I could do about those symptoms. All I could do was hope it would get better in time. I still have side-effects from the injury.

It would be more than a decade after the accident before I received a diagnosis. As it turned out, the neurologist missed the most common inherited neurological disorder, Charcot-Marie-Tooth syndrome, or CMT. I had all the classic symptoms.

Several years after my accident, my dad shared with me he had lost all feeling in his feet and could not climb stairs. The doctor told him it was a nerve disorder and not to worry about what it was called. His sister, my aunt, had a similar nerve disorder, too, so I knew it was genetic. Whatever it was that my dad had, I probably had it as well. Another piece of the puzzle.

Then an email came from my sister. It said "My girls have Charcot-Marie-Tooth (CMT)." I looked up the symptoms on the Internet and I knew I had it, too. Or at least I thought so.

Chapter 3
Genetically Gifted

You can't always choose the path you walk in life;
you can choose how you walk it.
—John O'Leary

On an early July afternoon in the 1950s, I entered the world with a number of genetic gifts, courtesy of Mom and Dad.

I can blame my being vertically challenged on both of them. My family is riddled with tiny woman on both sides of the family. When I met two of my mom's aunts, even though I was only 5 foot 2, I could see the tops of both of their heads when we were standing together to say goodbye. There is a family story about one of my great-grandmothers getting up on a stool to argue with her husband because she was so short.

From my dad, I got my analytical ability, asthma, and his Charcot-Marie-Tooth (CMT). It's only fair, since he got those same gifts from his dad, who got them from one of his parents. I had a 50:50 chance of getting CMT. I share CMT with his sister, my sister, and two nieces. Because my family has a mild case, I suspect at least two of my brothers have undiagnosed CMT. It is not uncommon for CMT to go undiagnosed.

Many medical professionals may see a line about CMT in a medical school book, but never recognize CMT or even see a CMT-affected patient.

The members of my family with CMT had classic symptoms all our lives. Rolling ankles, sprains, clumsiness, aches, fatigue, being cold, and poor handwriting were parts of our everyday life. As an athlete, I had tight calves and was always prone to injury. I was a puzzle to physical therapists. I did not have enough flexibility to walk correctly, much less run.

My dad built a first-floor bedroom when he retired at age 60 because he had no feeling in his feet and could no longer climb stairs. His doctor told him he had a genetic nerve disorder, but not to worry about what it was called. When my nieces were diagnosed with genetic testing, we finally knew the name of our ailment. We all had Charcot-Marie-Tooth.

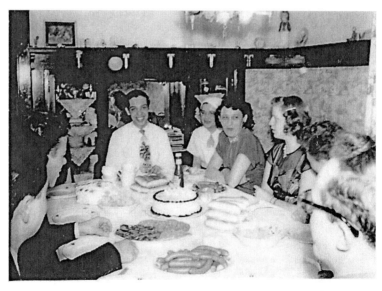

Dad is the handsome guy at the head of the table, with sister Elaine, mother-in-law May, and other family members.

I got my own diagnosis in August of 2010. It didn't seem right to me that no one has ever heard of CMT, even though 150,000 Americans have it. One in every 2,500 Americans is affected. That is as many people as have multiple sclerosis. There are 2.6 million with CMT worldwide.

My family's CMT symptoms were milder than most. I was still able to run, so I decided I had to do something to raise awareness about CMT; everyone has heard about MS, but it's very rare that anyone recognizes CMT.

One of the gifts I got from my mom is crazy determination and stubbornness. I prefer to call it being firm-minded. I have called on those traits over and over in my journey. I am especially determined when I feel I am righting a wrong.

Chapter 4
Why is Not the Right Question

A pessimist sees the difficulty in every opportunity;
an optimist sees the opportunity in every difficulty.
—Winston Churchill

When I looked up CMT symptoms on the Internet, I found a list of local doctors familiar with CMT. I made an appointment to see a CMT expert here in Milwaukee. When she said Charcot-Marie-Tooth, it was the first time I had heard it pronounced. I possibly had a disease I didn't even know how to pronounce. I hate those damned French words.

I was anxious for my answer. The doctor told me that while she was familiar with CMT, she specialized in rehab and did not usually diagnose. Since I was there, she said she would take a quick look. She ran me through a few quick strength, sensation, and range-of-motion tests that have since become so familiar. I remember one test was to put a tuning fork on my radial nerve, located at the base of the thumb. I really couldn't feel it. My hand hurt for the next 24 hours.

She said she was 90 percent sure I had CMT and referred me to a neurologist at a clinic where I was already a patient. Before I could be seen by a specialist, however, I had to get a referral from my primary physician. Of course, he was not familiar with CMT, but since I was a long-time patient, he was happy to give me a referral.

Referral in hand, I was off to another doctor She was interested in my case, because CMT is a bit rare. She said she might see one patient a year with CMT. In addition, my being an athlete with CMT added even more interest.

The full assessment took two days. She took a family history, which showed that my dad, aunt, sister, and two nieces with CMT. The general exam included tests for strength, balance, and sensation. The sensation test involves pricking your leg from the foot up; you tell the doctor when you can feel it. For me, it's almost to the knee.

Genetic tests can confirm CMT or you can have a nerve conduction velocity test and electromyography, or EMG. The EMG measures electric activity in the muscles. The nerve conduction test I had done once after my bike accident. It was just as much fun as the first time. For the test, electrodes are put on the arm, an electrical signal is run down the arm, and the time it takes for the signal to travel down the arm from one electrode to another is measured.

It takes twice as long for a signal to travel through the muscles in my arms as in an average person. My arm always jerks during this test. It is a most uncomfortable sensation to have an electrical signal passed down your arm. It's a test I hope I never have to have again.

All tests indicated I had CMT type 1A, the genetic family gift. I was actually relieved, for now I had the answer I had been seeking for years and the reason for all my symptoms, fatigue, and decreased athletic performance.

I never asked, "Why me? Why did I get CMT?" I realized my symptoms were mild compared to many people with CMT. I knew from reading about CMT how lucky I was to be running at all. I had always wondered why I had so much drive and discipline to work out, but was not blessed with an equal measure of athletic talent. I always had to work so hard at being an athlete.

I also think that God has a plan and purpose for everyone's life. You just have to be alert for the opportunity to use the gifts you have been given. I don't think God wanted me to have CMT, but I do think he gave me the wisdom to realize how lucky I was and the desire to do something to help. That is why I didn't think it was right to ask why.

In the book of Job, where God answers Job after all the troubles he went through. Job had lost his wealth, his children, and his health, and when Job questioned God, He responded with, "Where were you when I laid the foundations of the earth? ... To what are its foundations fastened?" In other words, God has wisdom and plans we may not understand, but He does have his plans and purposes. Even when things are difficult, God is right there beside us. My job was to discern God's will in my situation.

The right question was what would I do now, knowing what I knew about my CMT?

I felt blessed to be an athlete. Most people with CMT struggle to do simple tasks like button buttons, zip zippers, and open jars. Some struggle to turn keys in their cars or on the locks on their doors. Many use braces to walk and live with constant pain.

After my CMT diagnosis, I knew not only was I very blessed to be running; I needed to do something with it. What would I do with my ability to run? What would I do to make a difference?

My mom said many times when I was growing up, "To whom much is given, much is expected." I don't know if she was quoting John F. Kennedy or the verse from Luke 12:48. Either way, I always remembered it. So I felt I had a gift, a gift most people with CMT didn't have. What would I do with it?

My "what" was the Boston Marathon. I set the goal of running the Boston Marathon to raise awareness of CMT and to raise money for CMT research. I wanted to raise awareness because no one ever seemed to know about CMT. It did not seem right that so many people had a disease no one had ever heard of. I wanted to change that.

I knew a runner with CMT participating in the most prestigious marathon in the world would be a story worth telling. I could run and use my running to tell the story of CMT. The real question was, "How would I get into the Boston Marathon?"

Chapter 5
You Look Perfectly Fine

I can be changed by what happens to me.
But I refuse to be reduced by it.
—Maya Angelou

Late in 2012, I needed to find an assisted living residence for my dad. He'd been in a rehab nursing home for months and his time there was coming to an end. He had gone from being fairly independent to not being able to walk more than a few feet.

His CMT had accelerated overnight. He had to wear ankle foot orthotics (AFOs) for the first time. His balance was a mess and for the most part, he was confined to using a wheelchair. The therapists told us that it he likely would not be regain any more function.

The CMT severely limited the places we could place my dad because he needs two people to assist him. In addition, his care is much more expensive and we had very few options. It was all so heartbreaking because he felt really good and just wanted to go home.

The situation was also tough for me because I am most like my dad genetically. I share his CMT and asthma. I have the same problems swallowing. When I look at my dad, I see myself in 30 years. I am hoping being so active will slow the progression of my CMT and help me avoid my dad's fate. It is the only choice I have since there is no cure and no treatment. There is no way to slow progression.

During the course of finding an assisted living residence, I had to explain that my dad has CMT. Of course, no one had heard of the disease, so I educated the caregivers, explaining that it's genetic condition I share with several family members.

The representative from Senior Referrals told me, "You look perfectly fine." I cannot tell you how many times I have heard that. I know it is a common experience for anyone with a condition that isn't visible. While I know people mean well, if only they understood the experience of someone with one of these hidden limitations. I handed the rep a pen printed with my www.run4cmt.com website.

CMT is an invisible condition for many of us. I liken it to a house with termites, which looks perfectly fine from the outside, but is being eaten away from the inside. Everyone who thinks I look fine should pay my medical bills for one month. Staying healthy enough to be active with CMT is a constant battle. I am doing great, but I have challenges. I wish people who say I look fine could see me when I have to go to bed at 6 o'clock in the evening because I am so exhausted. It happens all the time.

No one has ever heard of CMT, but everyone knows about MS, I often explain that CMT is similar to MS. Not quite but it is a start to understanding and awareness of CMT. Charcot-Marie-Tooth disease, multiple sclerosis, and muscular dystrophy are three distinct problems within the body's neurological system.

CHARCOT-MARIE-TOOTH, MUSCULAR DYSTROPHY, AND MULTIPLE SCLEROSIS

Charcot Marie Tooth (CMT) is a disease of the body's peripheral nervous system. It gets its strange name from the three doctors who discovered it in 1886 (Jean Martin Charcot, Pierre Marie, and Howard Henry Tooth). CMT is also called "hereditary sensory and motor neuropathy." This means the disease is inherited or runs in families.

CMT causes problems with the sensory and motor nerves that run from the arms and legs to the spinal cord and brain. When the axons and myelin of the nerves become damaged, the messages running along the nerves move much more slowly or have a weak signal. Over time, this causes the muscles in the feet, legs, and hands to lose strength. This can happen unevenly, which can cause deformity as muscles waste away at different rates.

CMT affects an estimated 1 in 2,500 people in the United States or about 155,000 Americans. It affects 2.6 million people worldwide.

Cause
Charcot–Marie–Tooth disease is caused by mutations that result in neuronal proteins. Nerve signals are conducted by an axon with a myelin sheath wrapped around it.

Early Symptoms
- Clumsiness
- Slight difficulty walking because of trouble picking up the feet
- Weak leg muscles
- Fatigue

Common Symptoms

- Frequent tripping, ankle sprains, clumsiness and burning sensations in the hands and feet
- Foot drop- difficulty lifting the foot at the ankle
- Structural foot deformities; high arches and hammer toes
- Muscle wasting in the lower legs and feet
- Small muscles in forearms due to muscle wasting
- Weakness of the hips, legs, or feet
- Numbness or burning sensation in feet or hands
- Muscular atrophy in the hands causes difficulty with tasks involving manual dexterity such as writing, opening jars, closing zippers and buttons
- Loss of balance, tripping, and falling
- Poor tolerance for cool or cold temperatures. Many with CMT have chronically cold hands and feet
- Leg and hand cramps
- Difficulty grasping and holding objects
- Neuropathic pain (sometimes severe)
- Sleep apnea
- Accident prone (cut fingers, burn hands while cooking)
- Restless legs

Later Symptoms

- Similar symptoms begin to appear in the arms and hands
- Hand cramping
- Curvature of the spine (scoliosis)

Rarer Symptoms

- Speech and swallowing difficulties
- Breathing difficulties

- Hearing loss
- Vocal cord paralysis

Three-quarters of CMT patients report fatigue because it takes nerve signals twice as long to reach muscles. It is thought it takes twice the energy to do tasks.

Diagnosis

Because many doctors are not familiar with CMT, getting a diagnosis can be a challenge. These are the typical tests used to diagnosis CMT:

- **Medical and family history.** With most forms of CMT, you have a 50:50 chance to inherit if you have a parent with the condition. So a through family history is a good first step. My dad has CMT as did his dad and sister. I share the condition with several other family members.
- **Physical.** An examination is done to look for symptoms of CMT such as high arches, hammer toes, gait issues, etc. One of the tests is to prick the legs with a sharp object like a toothpick to see when you can feel it. The doctor gets almost to my knees before I start to feel the prick. Another test was to put a tuning fork to the nerve at the base of my thumb. I could not feel the vibrations, but my thumb hurt after the test for the next two days.
- **Nerve Conduction Velocity Test.** Electrodes are placed on the skin over the nerves on your legs and arms to measure how quickly the nerves carry electrical signals. I have had this test twice and I can tell you it was very uncomfortable for me. I hope I never have to have another one. My arm jumps when the signal gets to the end of my arm. My signal takes about twice the time as a non-CMT-affected person to travel the length of my forearm. In some places, the conduction is so slow they cannot get a signal.

- **Electromyography EMG).** A needle electrode is inserted through the skin over your legs and arms to measure electrical signals received by your muscles. The doctor warned me most of her patients hate her after this test because it can be so painful. I could not feel a thing. That just means I had lost quite a bit of sensation and function in the area.
- **Genetic Test.** A blood test may tell if you have CMT. The tests have come down a lot in price. The expense is lower if you know the type your family has. In my case it is CMT 1 A. My test was $600 and I had the test results in about a week.

Treatment

There is no cure for CMT and no drug therapies. Those with CMT, especially those with mild cases, can lead very active and full lives. Treatment may include one of the following:

- **Physical and Occupational Therapy.** Therapists work to improve muscle strength and stamina and to help people to be able to do the tasks of daily living.
- **Braces and orthopedic devices.** Custom shoes or shoe inserts help to improve walking ability. Leg braces prevent ankle sprains and improve walking ability
- **Surgery.** For some, surgery can help prevent or reverse foot and joint deformities.
- **Pain Management.** Pain drugs may be prescribed for those who have severe pain.

MUSCULAR DYSTROPHY (MD)

Muscular Dystrophy (MD) is a group of muscle diseases that weaken the musculoskeletal system and hamper locomotion. Muscular dystrophies are characterized by progressive skeletal muscle weakness, defects in muscle proteins, and the death of muscle cells and tissue.

The major forms of MD are Becker, limb-girdle, congenital, facioscapulo-humeral, myotonic, oculopharyngeal, distal, and Emery-Dreifuss muscular dystrophy. These diseases predominantly affect males, although females may be carriers of the disease gene.

Most types of MD are multi-system disorders with manifestations in body systems including the heart, gastrointestinal system, nervous system, endocrine glands, eyes and brain.

MD-affected individuals with susceptible intellectual impairment are diagnosed through molecular characteristics but not through problems associated with disability. However, a third of patients who are severely affected with DMD may have cognitive impairment, behavioral, vision and speech problems.

Symptoms
- Progressive muscular wasting
- Poor balance
- Drooping eyelids
- Atrophy
- Scoliosis (curvature of the spine and the back)
- Inability to walk
- Frequent falls
- Waddling gait

- Calf deformation
- Limited range of movement
- Respiratory difficulty
- Joint contractures
- Cardiomyopathy
- Arrhythmias
- Muscle spasms

Cause

These conditions are generally inherited, and the different muscular dystrophies follow various inheritance patterns. The most common cause of CMT (70-80% of the cases, CMT 1a) is the duplication of a large region on the short arm of chromosome 17 that includes the gene PMP22. CMT is divided into the primary demyelinating neuropathies (CMT1, CMT3, and CMT4) and the primary axonal neuropathies (CMT2), with frequent overlap.

Diagnosis

The diagnosis of muscular dystrophy is based on the results of muscle biopsy, increased electrocardiography, and DNA analysis. A physical examination and the patient's medical history will help the doctor determine the type of muscular dystrophy. Specific muscle groups are affected by different types of muscular dystrophy. Often, there is a loss of muscle mass (wasting), which may be hard to see because some types of muscular dystrophy, cause a build up of fat and connective tissue that makes the muscle appear larger.

Treatment

There is no known cure or treatment for any of the forms of muscular dystrophy. Physiotherapy, aerobic exercise, low intensity anabolic steroids, prednisone supplements may help to prevent contractures and maintain muscle tone. Orthoses (orthopedic appliances used for support) and corrective orthopedic surgery may be needed to improve the quality of life in some cases.

MULTIPLE SCLEROSIS (MS)

Multiple sclerosis (MS), also known as disseminated sclerosis, is an inflammatory disease in which myelin sheaths around axons of the brain and spinal cord are damaged, leading to loss of myelin and scarring. MS was first described by Jean Martin Charcot in 1886. He was one of the physicians who first described CMT as well.

Cause
The cause is not clear, but the underlying mechanism is thought to be either destruction by the immune system or failure of the myelin-producing cells. These changes affect the ability of nerve cells to communicate resulting in a wide range of signs and symptoms. It is more common in women and the onset typically occurs in young adults.

A person with MS can have almost any neurological symptom or sign, with visual, motor, and sensory problems being the most common. The specific symptoms are determined by the locations of the lesions within the nervous system, and may include:

- Loss of sensitivity
- Tingling, pins and needles feelings
- Numbness
- Muscle weakness
- Very pronounced reflexes
- Muscle spasms
- Difficulty in moving, coordination and balance.
- Problems with speech or swallowing.
- Visual problems
- Fatigue
- Acute or chronic pain

- Bladder and bowel difficulties
- Cognitive difficulties
- Depression or unstable mood.

Between attacks, symptoms may go away completely, but permanent neurological problems often occur, especially as the disease advances. Although much is known about the mechanisms involved in the disease process, the cause remains unknown.

There is no known cure for multiple sclerosis. Treatments attempt to return function after an attack, prevent new attacks, and prevent disability Life expectancy with MS is 5 to 10 years lower than that of an unaffected population About 2 to 150 per 100,000 people are affected.

Diagnosis
Multiple sclerosis can be difficult to diagnose since its signs and symptoms may be similar to other medical problems. The most commonly used diagnostic tools are neuro-imaging, analysis of cerebrospinal fluid and evoked potentials. Magnetic resonance imaging of the brain and spine shows areas of demyelization (lesions or plaques).

When I told one of my friends I had CMT, he asked me "What does it mean to have CMT?" I think he meant what did it mean to me? A good question because symptoms can vary so much even within families.

CMT affects me the most as an athlete. My dramatic decrease in performance after my bike accident was due to my CMT. I have spent years dealing with running injuries, like the stress fracture I got training from my first marathon. Physical therapists could never figure out why my calves were so tight and why I had so little flexibility in my ankles. Both are from the CMT.

When I race long distance, I get really bad blisters from my feet rubbing against my shoes because of the way I run due to the CMT. The blisters were so bad in my first marathon I bled through my shoes. In addition, my feet burn because of the nerve damage.

Many people report pain with CMT. I get pain in my legs if I go more than a day or two without working out. I often get pain in my hands. If I spend too long doing a chore, like painting or scraping, I will wake up the next day with loss of feeling in my hands. It takes about an hour to get the feeling back. I remember one day, my hands were numb almost the entire time during my 30-minute drive to work

If I overdo with gardening or working out, my whole body can feel like it is on fire, my legs get all jumpy, and my nerves just feel like they are frazzled.

I always seem to be tripping and dragging my feet. I'm not able to go for a hike without falling at least once.

In addition, I always seem to be cold. The one time of day I am warm is when I am in the hot tub at my health club or when I take a hot bath. My hands and feet are always cold.

CMT causes loss in manual dexterity, so for as long as I can remember, my handwriting has been terrible. My poor handwriting caused problems in school. I was pretty much a straight A student in grade school except for handwriting and gym. We had to practice our handwriting over and over, at least in the early grades. No matter how hard I tried, mine still came out sloppy. I also went to a Lutheran high school, where the teacher graded our notebooks and I got a D in high school German. When I took German in college, where no handwriting analysis was done, I got Bs.

The issues with my hands also affect my keyboard skills. I took typing in high school and got a much deserved D. I was not fast enough or accurate enough to do any better. It takes more time for me to acquire any motor skill and develop muscle memory. By the time I got to college, I could type 55 to 60 words per minute without too many errors.

As my CMT progresses, I am starting to lose my keyboarding skills. This means missing letters, because I don't always have the sensitivity in my hands to press hard enough on the keys. Being able to use a computer keyboard effectively is so important because all the work I do for my job is done via computer. If I lose my ability to type effectively, I will not be able to work.

The very worst thing about CMT is I am always tired—mind-numbing, worn-out exhausted. Every time I line up for a race or triathlon, I wonder where I will find the energy to finish.

For years, I searched for the answer to my constant fatigue. Since my childhood, I've had trouble falling and staying asleep. Some nights, I am awake all night. You cannot imagine how hard it is to go through life always tired. Sometimes I am so tired, I am not sure how I will get through the day. Sleep disturbances and fatigue are common with CMT.

My symptoms are milder than most with CMT. Many have difficulty walking without braces and live with constant fatigue and pain. They struggle to do simple, everyday tasks with their hands everyone else takes for granted.

I know I am so lucky that I can walk, even if I trip a bit, and even more lucky to be able to run and compete athletically.

Chapter 6
Why Boston?

*The marathon is a charismatic event. It has everything. It has
drama. It has competition. It has camaraderie. It has heroism.
Every jogger can't dream of being an Olympic champion, but
he can dream of finishing a marathon.*
—Fred Lebow, Co-founder of the New York Marathon.

Why did I choose the Boston Marathon as a goal race?
Of all the races and events I could do, why did I
pick that race?

There is no marathon more charismatic then the Boston
Marathon. It's known by runners simply as "Boston" and has
all the essential elements to make it a "must do" event. It is the
pinnacle racing experience. Boston has it all: tough course,
drama, competition, and raucous crowds.

The oldest annual marathon with the grandest tradition,
Boston is the Super Bowl of running events. It is on the "bucket
list" of any serious runner and is the only marathon with a time
standard for entry. To qualify for and run Boston is a crowning
achievement for any runner's career.

You get to run on the same course at the same time as the
best runners in the world. What other event has that?

You are looked with admiration by other runners. Even
non-runners know about the Boston Marathon. When you tell

people you are running Boston, they pay attention and have respect for you as an athlete.

The Boston Marathon was started in 1897 by the Boston Athletic Association (B.A.A.). The founding members wanted to re-create the Olympic Marathon they had witnessed the year before in Athens. The first race was 24.5 miles. In 1924, the race was lengthened to 26 miles, 385 yards to meet the new Olympic standard.

The race is always on the third Monday in April, Patriot's Day, to mark the ride of Paul Revere and the battles at Lexington and Concord. It's a state holiday in Massachusetts, giving lots of residents the day off and lending a party atmosphere to the course.

There 27,000 slots for this race. The exception was the 100-year anniversary in 1997, when the field was increased to 40,000. In 2010, entry spots to the race sold out in eight hours.

After 2010, a new rolling registration system was instituted. Runners must now register based on their qualifying times. The fastest runners register first, giving them a better chance at getting a spot in the race. It is not good enough just to run a qualifying time; you have to be among the best applying to gain a spot in the Boston Marathon. Qualification times were also tightened up. You need a faster time now to qualify than in past years.

To run Boston, you qualify by meeting the time standard for your gender and age group. For women in my age group (50-54), the time standard is 4 hours (4hrs00min00sec).

WOMEN'S QUALIFICATION TIMES FOR THE BOSTON MARATHON		
AGE MIN. MAX.		
18-34	3hrs 05min 00sec	3hrs 35min 00sec
35-39	3hrs 10min 00sec	3hrs 40min 00sec
40-44	3hrs 15min 00sec	3hrs 45min 00sec
45-49	3hrs 25min 00sec	3hrs 55min 00sec
50-54	3hrs 30min 00sec	4hrs 00min 00sec
55-59	3hrs 40min 00sec	4hrs 10min 00sec
60-64	3hrs 55min 00sec	4hrs 25min 00sec
65-69	4hrs 10min 00sec	4hrs 40min 00sec
70-74	4hrs 25min 00sec	4hrs 55min 00sec
75-79	4hrs 40min 00sec	5hrs 10min 00sec
80 and over	4hrs 55min 00sec	5hrs 25min 00sec

In addition, to qualify for Boston, you must run on a certified course before September of the year you apply. The course must be measured and certified by the United States Track and Field Association to prove they are of the stated length. Courses are certified for every distance from 1 mile to ultra-marathon. A course must be certified for a road performance to be accepted as a record.

How tough is it to get into Boston? I saw an article in a running magazine that said only 1 percent of Americans have completed a marathon. Many of the runners are not there to race but to experience and conquer a marathon. Anywhere from

8 to 20 percent of a marathon field will run a qualifying time. The race with the highest percentage of qualifiers at around 35 percent is the Boston Marathon. Boston runners can use the time from a previous Boston race to qualify the following year. Fewer women qualify than men. Age-group runners in the 18-34 range are the lowest percentage.

It is no longer enough to get a qualifying time. You must also get in. Registration is done on a rolling basis. The first to register are those at least 20 minutes under the qualifying time. The process then moves to runners closer to the qualification time until all slots are filled. Registration is all done on-line. You are not accepted until your qualifying race and time are verified.

When I ran my first marathon, the Lakefront Marathon in Milwaukee, the qualifying time for my age group was 3 hrs 50 minutes. I had missed the cut-off for Boston by ten minutes. It was not for lack of trying. I had such bad blisters, my feet bled through my running shoes. It was as painful as it sounds.

That first run would be my best effort. My next three marathons were 4:05, 4:15, and 4:20. The last two, I walked the last 6 miles and still finished with decent times. I wished I had trained harder.

In 2011, Geoffrey Mutai won Boston with a time of 2:03. He could run the course twice, take a shower, and be on a plane back to Kenya before I finished. The question was "How would I get in?" I knew I couldn't achieve the qualifying time needed because of my CMT. So what would I do?

Someone with CMT running Boston would be an achievement and a story worth telling. I wanted to show the

CMT community and the world what someone with this challenge can do. Finishing Boston would be the absolute best feeling in the world.

When I finished my first marathon, I felt there was not a thing in the world I couldn't do. Finishing a marathon has affected many aspects of my life. It gave me the confidence and determination to always keep going. Nothing can ever be tougher than those last few marathon miles. Fighting fatigue and mental demons as you struggle to finish gives you a strength that carries into all aspects of your life.

I knew Boston would be even more challenging. The course is legendary for its tough Newton hills. The most famous hill of all, known as "Heartbreak Hill," has been the demise of many runners.

The problem was getting in. I knew whatever way I found, it would not be easy. I did not even know if I could still run a marathon. I knew I couldn't achieve the qualifying time needed because of my CMT and the legacy of the bike accident, which caused an acceleration my CMT symptoms. I was so much slower than I once had been. Competing just did not seem fun anymore. So what could I do?

Chapter 7

The Boston Marathon—
Getting In

*A marathoner is a marathoner regardless of time. Virtually
everyone who tries the marathon has put in training over
months, and it is that exercise and that commitment, physical
and mental, that gives meaning to the medal, not just the day's
effort, be it fast or slow, It's all in conquering the challenge.*
—Mary R. Wittenberg, President New York Runners Club

E ntry to Boston is tough for most athletes. Even if you have a qualifying time, you aren't guaranteed entry. The qualifying times are tough and you have to be a pretty good athlete to be accepted.

So how would I get in? How would I achieve my Boston dreams? I searched the B.A.A. website looking for ways to get in because I knew there was no hope of meeting the regular women's time standard. Some of the options I considered were running for a charity, running with the American Athletic Medical Association, and other connections.

Charity
There are dozens of charities that have been awarded entry to the race. If you really want to run Boston but can't get in any other way, you can run for one of the charities, which are listed

on the Boston Marathon website. You have to apply and agree to raise at least $3,500 or more, depending on the charity. They actually take your charge card number and bill you if you don't raise the required amount. You have to apply through the charity itself. These spots fill up fast.

But I did not just want to run Boston—I wanted to represent CMT and run with a CMT charity. My main goal was to raise awareness for CMT. However, there were no CMT-related charities on the list.

To be accepted as a charity, you have to apply the year before the race. The charity must have an office in Boston or the New England area. New England charities with programming for kids are given priority, and preference is given to charities with programs in the greater Boston area.

I belonged to the Charcot-Marie-Tooth Association, CMTA, which did not qualify because it did not have a local Boston chapter. The Muscular Dystrophy Association was interested in applying, but the running team had to be managed by one person, which is time intensive. I thought it would be great if we could have runners represent some of the conditions under the MDA umbrella, but did not have time to recruit and manage a team. So charity options did not seem promising at that time.

American Athletic Medical Association

If you are a medical professional, such as a paramedic, nurse, or doctor, this is an option for participation. The American Athletic Medical Association runs a seminar just before the Boston Marathon. They also have a number of spots to run the

Boston Marathon because many of their members help with first aid on the course. They have a package for members to attend the seminar and run the marathon. In 2012, the cost was $1,500. Membership is around $50 for two years.

I considered this avenue because I'm a member of the National Ski Patrol and first responder. Plus I could run to raise awareness for CMT. Their spots sell out quickly as well.

Connections

There are eight small towns along the first ten miles of the Boston Marathon course. The B.A.A. gives each town entries into the race as compensation for the race coming through the community. This is a long shot, but if you have any connections with city officials in these towns, it might be possible to score a race bib. If you know a race official or member of the B.A.A., this might also be a way to get a number. At that time, I did not have connections in the greater Boston area, so using this line of attack wasn't an option.

I did have a friend who ran Boston in 2011. After that race, I went on line to check his results. Scrolling through the results, I noticed a division I had never heard of before: the "Mobility Impaired Division."

Athletes with Disabilities

Boston has an extensive program for wheelchair and visually impaired athletes. Local Milwaukee athlete Jean Driscoll has won the women's wheelchair division multiple times. However, this was the first time I had heard of the Mobility Impaired program. Doing my research, I found the following on the Marathon website:

> "Individuals with disabilities that affect their ability to ambulate may be granted the following extended qualifying times:
> The qualifying time is 6:00 hours for individuals who, because of the nature of their disability, have difficulty ambulating.
> The qualifying time is 8:00 hours for individuals who, because of the nature of their disability, need mobility aids such as prosthetics, leg braces or crutches to ambulate.
> All other individuals with disabilities must follow entry procedures and qualifying standards of either the B.A.A. or the established body.
>
> All individuals with disabilities must follow entry procedures and qualifying standards of the B.A.A. For persons with disabilities, the Boston Athletic Association follows the rules and guidelines of the International Paralympic Committee which are recognized by the International Stoke-Mandeville Wheelchair Sports Federation, Wheelchair Athletics USA, Disabled Sports USA and the United States Association for Blind Athletes. The Boston Marathon has push rim wheelchair and visually impaired/blind divisions, and a mobility impaired program. Medical documentation or proof of disability classification must be submitted with the entry form."

This was the lifeline I had been looking for. Would my CMT qualify me for this program? It was my only hope. I now had a goal to shoot for. To qualify for this program, I would need to make the six-hour time.

It had been over ten years since I had run long distance. I had stopped competing because after my bike accident. Because I did not understand why my performance had changed so much, I stopped competing out of frustration, It just was not fun anymore. I had gotten used to being a good athlete and when I wasn't anymore I decided to stop competing. However, I had never stopped running or training like I was going to race, for I wanted to be able to gear up quickly if I ever decided to do another marathon.

Could I even complete a marathon? I knew my CMT had progressed. Could I cover the distance and meet the time standard? Could I stay injury-free through the training? Would I even make it to the starting line? If I started, would I make it to the finish line? I didn't know, but I was about to find out.

Chapter 8
First Steps

Now bid me run and I will strive with things impossible.
—William Shakespeare

When I was diagnosed with CMT, I decided to dedicate my running to raising awareness of the disease and raising money for CMT research. I chose the Fox Cities Half-Marathon in September, 2010, as my re-entry race. A half-marathon is 13.1 miles, half the distance I would need to cover in a full marathon.

I called the Charcot-Marie-Tooth Association (CMTA) to ask about raising funds. The national CMTA newsletter was always urging members to do some type of event to raise money for CMT research. Some members had fundraising pages on their websites. Many were family members of those affected with CMT and many were doing runs to raise money. However, no CMT-affected athletes were raising funds with races. When I talked to the fundraising coordinator, he said he only knew of one other CMT-affected athlete, a triathlete living in England. I was beginning to understand that being a long-distance runner with CMT was a bit unusual.

The CMTA helped me set up a fundraising page. My initial diagnosis was in May, and when I got confirmation of my CMT in August, I had already started training for the half-marathon.

I had never stopped running, and ran three days a week, including an hour-long run on weekends. I still loved the activity and the feeling running gave me, especially when I wasn't measured against others in a race.

My usual routine was to do a speed workout, tempo run, and long run each week. Every three weeks, I cut the workouts in half do give my body a rest. This is the same pattern I used to train for my marathons.

The Fox Cities Half-Marathon starts in Menasha and ends in Neenah, along the shores of beautiful Lake Winnebago. This race would be a test to see if I could still run long distance. I wondered if my CMT had progressed to where it was not possible to run a half or full marathon, and needed to know that before committing to Boston.

It was my first fund-raising and awareness event. I hadn't run a race in six years.

* * * * *

I quit racing after a 5K evening run in June in Pewaukee, Wisconsin. The race was one more reminder of the many ways the accident had affected my running.

Throughout the race, my feet burned and hurt. I could not seem to get times better than 10-minute miles. If I couldn't be competitive, I did not want to compete. In road races, every runner wears a watch so you know your time per mile since every mile on the course is marked. Speed workouts are also done on quarter-mile tracks so when runners do speed workouts on these tracks, they are timed as well.

My work schedule had also changed. I was working a rotating shift, sometimes 2nd shift until midnight once a month and one Saturday and Sunday each month. My job was working as a supervisor in the distribution dispatch center of our local utility. We dispatched personnel any time there was a problem on the electric system. We also dispatched crews to repair damage done by storms. Since storms are not scheduled my work days were often long and unpredictable. That schedule made it hard to get to races. I've never been a morning person and could just not get up to run a morning race after working until midnight.

* * * * *

When I started training for the 2010 half-marathon, I went to a sports medicine clinic to get some help with my running gait. They did a video analysis of me running on a treadmill. When the therapist and I looked at my stride, you could clearly see my running was not normal.

CMT had most affected my right side. My right leg swings from the hip to clear the foot drop caused by the CMT. The foot drop is caused by muscle weakness caused by nerve damage.

The therapist worked with me to change the way I ran. This was a real challenge for someone with my condition because leg muscles are also weakened by the CMT. He checked with the lead physical therapist to find out if there were any exercises for runners with CMT. The head of physical therapy for the largest sports medicine clinic in the area told my therapist that she thought people with CMT couldn't run!

This meant that as far as I knew at the time, I was breaking ground. The first therapist after my diagnosis specialized in nerve disorders. He knew about CMT, but when he did a search on exercise and CMT, he did not find anything.

* * * * *

Before I set up my fundraising page for the CMTA, I checked with the Fox Cities Half-Marathon race director. The purpose of the run was to raise money for the local hospital. I wanted to be sure it was OK to use the race to raise money for my charity. They gave me the go-ahead. I sent out fundraising letters to all my friends and family, asking for a dollar donation for the race.

When I spoke with the race organizers, I also learned that they were holding a contest to determine the "Most Inspiring Women" of the race. Participants were asked to tell their individual stories and winners would be awarded special pink race singlets. To my surprise, I was selected as one of the "Most Inspiring Women" of the race and I wore my special pink singlet proudly on race day.

Because Menasha is about two hours from Milwaukee, I booked a hotel to stay overnight to be well-rested the following day.

Everything went smoothly pre-race. I found my hotel and visited the expo. Every big race seems to have an expo where local vendors sell running-related items and medical providers offer their services. Race packet pick-up was also at the expo. You pick up your number, tee shirt and timing chip. The chip records your progress along the course and your finish time.

I did not sleep at all the night before the race. I was so nervous. I knew this would be a big test.

I arrived at the start hours early. The one glitch in the day was that the radio I had purchased just days before decided not to work. .Music had accompanied me on every previous race and I wondered how I would get through the race without it.

Early fall days can be chilly in Wisconsin and the temperature was in the upper 30s when the gun went off. It would not get much above 40 degrees all day. Actually, those cool temperatures are great for a long race. About half way in, my feet started to burn and hurt, which could have signaled the start of a blister. A short time later, it started to rain, but the drizzle stopped after a few minutes.

Even though I did not have music, I watched the other runners and listened to the entertainment scattered along the course. By the end, I hurt and was tired, but I had done it! Thirteen miles—Menasha to Neenah—in 2 hrs and 12 minutes.

After the race, I took a shuttle back and got off when the bus stopped in an industrial park. I didn't know there was more than one shuttle stop and as it turned out, I was miles away from my car back in Menasha. I mentioned what happened to two ladies who got off the bus at the same time, and they offered to take me back to my car. I love Wisconsin people. Not only will they help, but you can trust them when they do.

It turned out that they were from Clintonville, a small town just 15 miles from where my dad lives. One woman was the race director of a triathlon I had done two weeks earlier. We chatted like old friends and in about 15 minutes, they had me back to my car.

Now that I knew I could do a half-marathon, it was time to pick out a marathon to try and qualify for the Mobility Impaired Division of Boston.

The only disappointment from the half-marathon were my fundraising efforts. Not one of my brothers or sister contributed, nor did my mom. I was shocked and hurt by their response.

Chapter 9
The Sounds of Silence

Silence is a true friend who never betrays.
—Confucius

S ilence can be a welcome break from the rush and noise of
the day. I love coming home to a quiet house. I have
always enjoyed long periods of solitude to reflect and
refresh. Most of us are uncomfortable with silence and try to
fill every void in conversation.

Part of my job is interviewing job candidates. One of the
techniques I use is to sit quietly as an answer is given. Candidates often keeping talking and disclose information they might
not otherwise do because they are not comfortable with silence.

Watch most runners and you will see an iPod or radio that
provides the sound track for their workout. Most Americans
"need" the constant background noise of TV or music.

As a long-distance runner, I am used to long periods of
time alone. I don't use music to train. I've gotten comfortable
with the sounds of nature and my own breathing being the only
sounds I hear.

Silence can also be a form or rejection. The partner or
friend giving you the "silent treatment" out of anger is familiar
to all of us.

Silence and rejection were not the expected responses when I began to disclose my CMT and raise money. They took me by surprise. It hurt and sometimes made me angry. What really puzzled me was the silence from my immediate family and some really long-time friends.

I had a group of girlfriends from high school. We lost touch after school when they got married and raised their families. At a reunion, we all reconnected and it was like we had never been apart. These friends from my youth made me laugh. I thought they would always be in my life. For years, we got together for dinner every few weeks and even did girls' weekends. I got emails from each of them almost every day, mostly just that silly stuff people pass around the Internet.

After I sent out my fundraising letter, which also announced my CMT, I almost never heard from two of them again. I got a sympathy card from one when my mom died and that is all I have heard. I get a Christmas card once a year. Neither of them has ever asked about my CMT or expressed any sympathy. It is as if it never happened.

One of my high school friends has stood by me. Maybe it is because she has family members with autism and understands the value of friends when things in life happen.

I was hurt by the silence from my brothers and sister. Not one of them even asked about the CMT. My sister has it and so do two of her girls. One brother even rudely put the letter aside as I handed it to him. He pleaded poverty, even though he had been on two trips to Asia in the past year to visit his girlfriend.

My dad grudgingly gave $10 after I spent $10 buying lottery tickets for his Lion's Club raffle, tickets I have been buying every year for years. When I told him the money was for CMT research, he asked how long before there would be a cure. When I told him 10 to 15 years, he shrugged his shoulders and said, "What do I care? It will be too late for me."

I think I would have gotten a more positive response if I had been asking for money for some random fundraiser. Are they embarrassed? Do they think I am doing OK? I know it isn't cancer or ALS, but I have it. Don't they care? Should they be even a little interested just because I was doing it? Even a bit of polite interest would have been acceptable.

Silence tells me nothing. It has made me question my relationship with each one of them. Did they not even care enough to ask a question or make a casual remark? Do they care about how I am doing or what it means to me to have CMT? I can understand "no" in a tough economy. I understand the need to pay bills and make tuition payments. I can understand being busy and forgetting to give.

I did get great support from friends and extended family when I sent out my first fundraising letter. I was so touched by a friend who is a single mom; she apologized because she could only give $5. I was touched by her generous heart and desire to help. I had several friends who were really curious about CMT and how it affected me personally.

It is also hard when I send in a request for sponsorship or submit an article for publication and I hear nothing. "No" I understand. "No" has certainty. With silence, I wonder if the request had even been received.

Since that first half-marathon in 2010, some of my family members have begun to support me. My oldest brother was at the finish line when I ran the Madison Marathon to qualify for Boston. My brother and his wife in Texas have supported to my fundraising efforts and have watched me compete twice in Austin at the National Paratriathlon Championships. My older brother has given now several times to my fundraisers as well. My sister still has never made a donation, even though her two daughters have this disease. However, her ex-husband has been very generous in his support. I have two other brothers that have never given anything or ever even asked about my CMT.

Here is what this silence has taught me. I can't take the lack of response personally. I believe my mission is to raise awareness of CMT. If I make a request, I have made someone aware of CMT. The rest is up to God. If He means for them to be part of my work, He will have them respond. Jesus told his disciples that if they went to a town and were not welcome, to leave and shake the dust from their sandals. In other words, don't take it personally and move on. If someone wants to give or be part of raising awareness, that is up to God and it's not about me. God may have something else in mind for them and me.

Chapter 10
Guys in Shirts

Use what talents you possess, the woods will be very silent if no birds sang there except those that sang best.
—Henry Van Dyke, American author and educator

Every elite athlete seems to have a corporate sponsor. Bike racers, runners, skiers, golfers, and snowboarders all seem to have uniforms with the logos of their sponsor companies. It would definitely be cool to be a sponsored athlete.

The coach leading a swim class I took in Milwaukee is a triathlete sponsored by Zoot. Sponsored athletes always seemed to be successful and talented. In Milwaukee, local running stores recruit the best runners to race for them. These athletes get to wear the team uniform as a mark of their athletic prowess. The closest I ever got to one of those uniforms was dating a local elite runner.

Actually, I don't even have much experience being on a team. I played volleyball in 7th and 8th grade and sat the bench for two years. I did not get into even one game. It seems I just don't have the talent to ever be sponsored, even by a local running store.

* * * * *

To help me get ready for the Madison marathon I had chosen to qualify for Boston, I decided to race in a local 10K running series of five races. Of course, the local teams were all there, including the team sponsoring the event, the Racers Against Childhood Cancer (RACC), which has running, bike, and triathlon teams. They raise an impressive amount of money for cancer research. Each of their members also commits to raising a certain amount of money each year.

I was joined by my college friend and roommate, Cheryl Monnat. Cheryl first got me into competition and was there to encourage me when I re-entered the racing world. It was nice to have a friend along for the races. It made running a lot more fun.

Cheryl had also set a goal of running a local fall marathon in hopes of qualifying for Boston. Doing the 10-K series would help her as she prepared to train for her first marathon. Once you get to the 20-mile mark, you can tell yourself, "It's just a 10K now."

When I race, all my competitive juices kick in. I love passing people and push myself to get the best time possible. It isn't easy. I remember getting to the half-way point and thinking "God, couldn't you find something easier for me to do?"

While I was running the first race of the series, I passed several men wearing the RACC uniform. I thought, "Wow, they're just guys in shirts. I'm faster than they are. We can be 'guys in shirts,' too." Thus was born the idea for Team CMT.

I decided I would start a team to raise awareness of CMT. That way, runners and everyone along the course would see our uniforms and learn about CMT. I thought it would be a great idea to ask family members of those affected with CMT to join us.

That was in January. It took a bit of time to get the logo for our first design, then there was a slight problem with the shirt order. We finally made our debut on April 30th, 2011. Friends Cheryl Monnat, Robert Kearney, and I ran the first race, a 10K in Brown Deer, Wisconsin. Cheryl took first place in her age group and I took second.

I wrote an article for the CMTA newsletter asking athletes to join our team. To my surprise, people from all over the country asked to join. Many of them were runners, cyclists, and triathletes affected by CMT. We used the CMTA STAR (Strategy to Accelerate Research) logo. So our shirts—white racing singlets—said Team CMT and STAR in navy blue. I

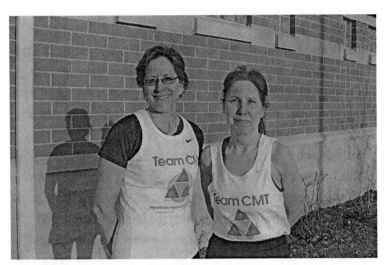

The author and friend Cheryl Monnat in the Team CMT singlet.

liked being a star. Our singlets had a very professional and classic look. We were "big time" now, just like all the other teams. I paid for all the costs associated with the uniforms.

CMTA's involvement was to let us use the logo and we raised funds for them. Later, we repeated the process all over again when we joined the Hereditary Neuropathy Foundation (HNF). This time, the HNF paid for the uniforms, making us genuine "officially sponsored athletes.

We may not be the fastest runners, but there are things more important than talent—like running to raise awareness of CMT. What we lack in talent, we make up for in determination and perseverance.

It was really nice to be competing again. This time, I was running for a cause and not just for medals. It was even more exciting to me hearing from family members and CMT-affected athletes from all over the country. Most people with CMT have never met anyone with CMT outside their own families. They may never have known another athlete with the same struggles. It has been really exciting to get to know them and share in their accomplishments and excitement in finding and joining the team.

Chapter 11

How Many Steps in a Marathon?

"Why couldn't Pheidippides have died at 20 miles?
—Frank Shorter, marathon gold medalist, 1972 Summer Olympics.

Imagine having to pay attention to every step you take during a run. Imagine being at the starting line, wondering when the burning and blisters will start. Imagine not knowing if your feet will cause you to stumble or trip.

This is what I face as an athlete every time I walk to the starting line. I also face fatigue before I race one step. Imagine being at the starting line so tired you wonder how you will run one mile, much less an entire race.

Because of my CMT, I have high arches and a very prominent ball of my foot. When I land on my foot, there is a twist in my stride as I push off on the ball of my foot each and every time I take a step. The burning is from CMT nerve damage. The fatigue is also due to nerve damage. It takes twice as much energy for someone with CMT to do everyday tasks, so think about the energy it takes for my muscles to run a marathon.

Since I have foot drop, there is the risk of tripping every time I take a step. I have to pay attention to every step. Foot drop is kind of a funny term. It is caused by the CMT, because the muscles in the lower legs get weak and very tight. The foot basically flops forward. To walk, your ankle needs to flex about six degrees as your foot rolls through a walking or running motion. The foot drop means my foot often catches as I walk or run. This can cause tripping or means my foot doesn't completely roll through the running motion. It is like having a little brake that slows my running motion with every step.

Those were the challenges I faced as I ran my marathon to qualify for Boston: the Madison Marathon in May 2011.

I had one shot since application for Boston 2012 started September 1, 2011, which meant I had to run a qualifying time on a Boston-certified course.

A marathon is 26 miles 385 yards. It was one of the events at the first modern Olympics in 1896 in Athens. The length of that marathon was 25 miles. I wish they had left it there. The distance was increased to the present distance for the London Olympics in 1908—so the royal children could see the finish of the race from their palace balcony.

According to legend, the marathon had its origins in ancient Greece. The messenger Pheidippides ran from the plains of Marathon to deliver the message of victory by the Greeks over the Persians. He ran the distance and dropped dead. Not a good start for the history of the race.

The 26.2 mile distance is 1,660,032 inches. With each stride, I move 30 inches, so it will take me 55,334 steps to go the distance. If Pheiddipedes had stopped at 20 miles, he would have saved me lots of steps.

I took the race one step at a time. There will be many times I will want to stop. The last 6 miles are always the hardest. The body is fighting fatigue and that voice inside the head asking "What on earth are you doing to me?"

In Madison, I will line up at the starting line, ready to take 5,745 steps. Can't wait to get to the last one as I cross the finish line. When I cross, I hope to have my Boston qualifying time.

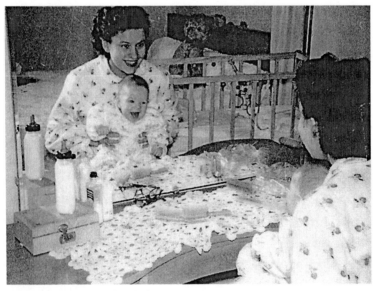

Mom, Maryanne Karl (Wodke)

Chapter 12
Marathon Dedication:
For Mom

I run because it is so symbolic of life. You have to drive
yourself to overcome the obstacles. You might feel that you
can't. But then you find your inner strength, and you realize
you are capable of so much more than you thought.
—Arthur Blank, co-founder of Home Depot

Every time I run a marathon, I dedicate the run to
someone. It helps me to get thorough the race when
things get tough.

My first race I ran for my nephew Brandon. He'd sent me
a paper Flat Stanley doll as part of a middle school project. I
pinned Flat Stanley to my running number. Flat Stanley made
the entire distance in just under four hours. When Flat Stanley
returned to his owner, he took my finisher medal from the Lake
Front Marathon with him. I dedicated other races to various
nieces and nephews.

The Madison Marathon will be no different. That race
will be special since I have three Team CMT members running
in the half-marathon with me; it is my first marathon since my
diagnosis. It is the race I will use to qualify for Boston. I am
dedicating the Madison Marathon to my mom, who passed
away in March of 2011.

For her last year, my mom was in and out of hospitals and nursing homes. It was a real challenge to sneak in marathon training around visits. She had dementia, so she knew nothing about CMT and my work to raise awareness. I hoped she would be pleased and proud. I intend to run a good race on Sunday in her honor.

* * * * *

My mom 's dementia made her a difficult patient. She often thought she was not being fed or otherwise taken care of. She would plead for me to let her go home because she had not had anything to eat or drink all day. I knew it wasn't true because I was often there when her tray was brought. She gave caregivers a hard time as well and they always dealt with it in a patient and loving way.

Often I would go to visit, only to be kicked out by her because I would not get her released from the place she thought was keeping her prisoner. That behavior was not my mom; it was the dementia. I went to the hospital or nursing home almost every day just to make sure she was being well cared for. If I did not talk to her, I touched base with her nurses for a report.

Several times over the last couple years of her life, my siblings and I thought we going to lose her only, to see her bounce back.

On a Thursday in March, I went to see her. It was the same day Elizabeth Taylor died. I remember my mom telling me, she was mad at God. She was ready to die and she felt like she was better. A voice told me to sit and stay. I recognized this just might be the surge some people get right at the end and I told her so. She seemed to like that and got comfort from it.

We must have talked for over two hours. We talked about Elizabeth Taylor, old movies, and all kinds of ordinary things. We also talked about some really important stuff, like all the details she wanted me to know about her funeral. There was truly no need to tell me, since she had written it all out for me in her beautiful handwriting. Her funeral was important to her and I let her go over all the details. I could give her peace by assuring her it would all be taken care of. She told me to get my brothers to come, that she wanted to see them.

After hours of talking, I was exhausted. As I left, I hugged her hard and told her I loved her. She said good-bye and that she would see me in Heaven. I stopped and looked at her and told her to get a place ready for me. She said she would, one with gardens and Golden Retrievers, both things she loved.

It was hard to leave. That was the last real conversation I had with my mom. By the next night, she had slipped back into her dementia and passed away a few days later.

For the few hours my mom's dementia had lifted, I had my "old" mom back. She had been hard of hearing for years, but there was no trouble with her hearing that night. I got a rare gift—the chance to say good-bye. How many people wish they'd had that opportunity? It was such a blessing. She was so tired, she was ready to go, and I was ready to let her go. I knew she was with the Lord she loved so much.

There isn't a day I don't think about my mom. She was an old-fashioned, cookie-baking, PTA-attending, dinner-on-the-table-every-night mom. When I was in high school, she got up every morning and made me breakfast before my 6 a.m. bus. When I wanted to go to a private high school, my stay-at-home mom got a job to pay the tuition. When I was in the grade school musical, my mom—who hated sewing—made me a beautiful costume.

Mom never learned to ride a bike, but she encouraged me to be active. Her parents did not allow her to attend college, but she made sure I got the chance for an education. She loved to cook and we spent hours together cooking, baking, and sharing recipes. For her, food equaled love. You could not be in her house more than a few minutes without being offered something to eat. We both shared a love of gardening and she would proudly show me her garden whenever I visited. Mom also had a deep belief in God that gave her strength. She instilled that faith and strength in me as well.

My mom was feisty right to the end and faced death bravely. I will take that same courage with me as I run. I hope I made her proud as I ran the Madison Marathon in her honor.

Chapter 13
We're All Cowards

I have the same doubts as everyone.
Standing on the starting line, we're all cowards.
—Alberto Salazar, winner of three consecutive New York marathons
and the 1982 Boston Marathon

would never have thought a world-class runner would feel the same fear I feel as a middle-of-the pack participant. Well, middle- to back-of-the-pack actually.

As I lined up for the Madison Marathon that Sunday in May, I wondered if I had done the right training. Had I run long enough? Had I pushed enough in my tempo runs? Had I gotten enough rest days? Had I done the right cross-training? Had I eaten the right stuff? Had I raced enough? Had I pushed myself too much? Will I make it? Can I handle the pain and fatigue I know will be my friends for a large part of the race?

A thousand questions crossed my mind. I never dreamed that every runner toeing the line had the same doubts and fears. My fears weren't from not knowing what to expect. Madison would be my fifth marathon. I knew the physical endurance and mental toughness that are needed to finish. I knew the pain and exhaustion to expect. What I didn't know was if I could do it again. I wondered if I was up to it one more time. Would I quit?

My CMT provides me with a built-in excuse to quit. I wonder how my feet will hold up. During my first marathon, my feet blistered so badly they bled through my shoes. The pain from my quads was intense. The CMT means I don't have enough flexibility in my calves to walk decently, much less run.

As a result of work with my physical therapist, I changed my running gait this year. I had been running on my toes, and switched to landing on my heels and rolling up in hopes of having a more efficient and pain-free run. The change meant I now had sore and tired hamstrings. How will they hold up on race day? Will the change work? I won't know until I run the race.

The race is 26 miles. Twenty-six miles is a long way to drive, much less run. Will I have the energy to run the entire race? It has been ten years since I ran my last marathon and I am not sure what to expect once I get past the half-way point. Will I make it? After I ran the Fox Cities Half-marathon, I was so tried and my feet were so sore, I did not know how I would run 13 more miles to do a full marathon. Could I still do it and could I do it fast enough to qualify for Boston?

Another member of Team CMT would run the half-marathon that day. She likes to know every twist, turn, and elevation on the course. She let me know two weeks before the race, the first half is hilly and there is a large hill in the last mile of the marathon. Me, I like to be surprised. It keeps the experience interesting

I also have the added pressure and expectations of being part of Team CMT. I was blogging several times a week about my quest to qualify for the Boston Marathon.

Everyone who knew me would want to know about the race. But this experience was no longer about me. My fears and challenges did not matter. My goal was no longer a personal best time or a medal. Those were out of reach anyway. The goal was now to raise awareness of CMT. I had a bigger purpose and goal to drive me to the finish line. I had to prove to the Boston Athletic Association that I could run a marathon in 6 hours to qualify for the mobility-impaired division. I knew that running a high-profile event like the Boston Marathon would be a great way to raise awareness. Being a runner with CMT running in Boston would be a dynamic story I could use to gain publicity for our cause.

Strangely, those considerations did not lessen my pressure or fear. To be accepted to Boston would mean a huge stage for raising awareness of CMT. I run for all those with CMT who can't. I run so when they tell someone they have CMT, they don't get a blank look. Imagine having a disease that robs you of the use or your hands or legs and no one has ever heard of it. I run for all of us with CMT. I run because it's a miracle I can run at all.

"The whole enchilada" rested on the race I would run in Madison. I had to get a qualifying time by September 1st and it was already the end of May. If I failed in Madison, It was doubtful I could train for and run another marathon to meet the deadline.

I was going to give it my best shot despite every fear and limitation. Along with the fear and limitations I also have an insane stubbornness and determination. I was willing to do whatever it took to get there.

Chapter 14
None Tougher

*That was without a doubt the hardest physical thing
I've ever done.*
—Lance Armstrong, after finishing the New York Marathon

Bicyclist Lance Armstrong won seven straight *Tour de France* races, including numerous stage races in the mountains, yet in his own words, the New York Marathon had been the toughest race he ever faced.

After running the Madison Marathon, I couldn't agree more. I had to fighter harder for this finisher medal than I had for any of the other four marathons in which I've completed.

I had been fighting some kind of virus all month with sore throat, headache, and ear pain. The day of the race, I woke up with nausea and couldn't eat more than half a protein bar for breakfast.

I hadn't slept much the night before, which is pretty common if the conversations at the starting line were the average experience. It was going to be a long day and there was a good possibility I wouldn't finish. I also knew this was my one shot this year—or maybe ever—to qualify to run the Boston Marathon.

Sometimes you feel kind of tired at the start of a race, but your training takes over and you get into a rhythm. That didn't happen for me in Madison. This race was tough from the start and every mile was a struggle.

The course was one hill after another. I finished the first six miles in about an hour. I felt like I was finished at 13 miles and promised myself I would walk if I made it to 20 miles. I hit the 20-mile mark at 3:30, three and a half hours. As I hit the 20-mile mark, it started to rain. I ran the last 6 miles in the rain.

I just wasn't physically or mentally tough enough to keep going. I walked the next mile and then did a combination of running and walking to complete the race in 4:51:28, four hours and fifty one minutes. I was lucky to finish on a day when physically, it just wasn't happening for me. I was totally wrecked at the end. The whole race had been run on guts, determination, and a lot of prayer.

Still, the finish put me at 15 out of 24 women in my age group. I wonder where I would have placed with that 4:30 finish. More importantly, I had finished well under the six hours needed to qualify as mobility impaired runner for Boston. I know I will do better next time.

Whether I am accepted to run the Boston Marathon in 2012 was now in the hands of the Boston Athletic Association. Like any other runner, I will apply when registration opens and hope for the best.

I can't help but reflect about the marathon I had run ten years before. I had walked the last six miles and still finished at 4:20, four hours and twenty minutes. The difference in my finish times between then and now showed me how much I had lost in strength and speed.

As the CMT progresses, I will lose more. This really might be my last shot to run Boston.

After a brief rest, in July, I returned to training for my next marathon; the Marine Corps Marathon in Washington D.C. on October 29th. No pressure to qualify with this one. I had signed up for this race in case I did not qualify in Madison. My time for Marine Corps can be used for the 2013 Boston Marathon.

The Marine Corps Marathon is a bit of insurance. If I don't get into Boston with my Madison Marathon race, I will try again with hopefully a qualifying time from Marine Corps. It is also a good opportunity chance to raise awareness of CMT. The course is lined with 100,000 spectators. Lots of them will get to see our Team CMT uniform. Two Team CMT members will be running: me in the marathon and Cheryl Monnat in the 10K. I can't wait!

Chapter 15

Marine Corps Marathon Dedication

I run because I can,
When I get tired, I remember those who can't run.
What they would give to have this simple gift I take for granted
and I run harder for them.
I know they would do the same for me.
—Unknown

When Team CMT member Joyce Kelly contacted the national CMTA about starting a running team, she was told people with CMT don't run. More than one physical therapist believes people with CMT can't run. Well, some of us can and I set out to prove it one more time at the Marine Corp Marathon.

Marathons are tough. I dedicated the Madison Marathon to my mom. The Marine Corps Marathon is dedicated to the members of Team CMT. Here is what I wrote to the members:

I am dedicated this race to the athletes of Team CMT. First to my teammates who have CMT. Many of you were told not to run, but you did it anyways. CMT makes us slow and presents challenges, but it can't keep us from the sports we love. Joyce, Jude, Jess, Jane, Richard, Michael,

Donna, Erika, Cody, Dale and Tosha, you inspire me. When I get frustrated about being slow and complain about injuries, you all remind me how lucky we are to still be running.

To all the Team CMT members running for family members; Bill, Karen, Kathy, Pam, Dawn, Gary, Tashua, Megan, Charlie, Tim, Alyssa, Shirley, Ruth, Will, Shelia and Emmalee. Thanks for your support and your willingness to raise awareness for your family members. It means more to us then we can possible say.

Finally to all the other Team CMT members who are running just because one of us asked you to help, Cheryl, Robert, Katie, Morgan, Tony, David, Paul, Gloria, Brett, Scott, Jim, Kevin, Kim, Ruth, Glydnis, and Anthony. Some of you I haven't ever met, but you stepped forward when one of us asked. What a true act of love. Your kindness means more than I can say.

My teammate Cheryl will also be running. She was my very first team member. She listened patiently as I talked on and on about forming this team and listened to my ideas for singlet designs. She continues to be one of our most ardent supporters. She has been with me for virtually every race and will be running the 10 K on Sunday and providing moral support. Thanks Cheryl!!

I will be running for all of you, doing what many of us have been told is impossible. We aren't supposed to exercise too hard and definitely not to run marathons. Sunday will be tough because I am fighting a couple injuries. But it won't be impossi-

ble because I will be carrying the good wishes, hopes and faith of Team CMT with me. Thanks Guys! The finisher medal at the end is always sweet. This time it will be even better. There are expected to be 100,000 spectators on the course. We will be doing a lot of awareness raising with this race. See you at the finish!.

* * * * *

The August before the Marine Corps Marathon, Cheryl and I ran the Reykjavik half-marathon in Iceland. We based ourselves in an apartment right off the main shopping avenue and did day trips the week before the race. We stayed near the harbor and got to train on the course before the race. Reykjavik is really a wonderful city and I enjoyed my visit. I felt like a native after a week of exploring the island..

Iceland has volcanic landscape and tremendous water-falls. I had hoped to see a puffin when I was there and on one of our day trips, we got within feet of dozens of them and took in sites like the Blue Lagoon.

Cheryl and I finished the week with the half-marathon. There were runners from all over Europe. When I run, I like to talk to other runners. I saw two young ladies in identical pink shirts. I asked if they were on the same team and it turned out they were Danish sisters. They asked me where I was from and I told them Milwaukee. I heard a shout from behind me from another runner from Milwaukee. It really is a small world.

The weather for the race could not have been more perfect. It was 60F and sunny. The course was flat and fast.

Cheryl and I both had good times and a great experience. The race entry included free entry into one of the local swimming pools heated with geothermal water.

A big festival started right after the race. Iceland has a population of 300,000, about one third of whom live in Reykjavik, the rest come to town for the festival. It is a mixture of cultural festival and street fair all rolled into one. In addition to plays and showings at art galleries, roving performers and street concerts provided entertainment. Food vendors were set up all over the center of the city. The evening ended with fireworks at midnight. The day just happened to be Cheryl's birthday. It was a great day to celebrate her special day and a great race—a fitting end to our stay in Iceland.

* * * * *

I like doing at least one destination event a year. It is fun to explore a new location then run a race. By the time I run the race, I feel like a local. So I looked forward to another great destination race in Washington DC. I love history and museums. Washington is full of those.

Chapter 16
The Marine Corps Marathon

There will be days when I' don't know if I can run a marathon;
there will be a lifetime knowing that I have.
—Unknown

I don't like big events and have avoided big races like Al's Run in Milwaukee. Al's Run is named after former Marquette coach Al McGuire. He led Marquette University to the NCAA basketball Championship in 1977. This run is a community event drawing 30,000 runners to the streets of Milwaukee to raise money for Children's Hospital. The Marine Corps Marathon was predicted to draw 30,000 runners and 100,000 spectators. I couldn't resist the chance to raise awareness on such a big stage by running the event.

The Marine Corps Marathon has a reputation of being a well-organized and fun race and this year, it didn't disappoint. It is a relatively flat course that goes around the Capitol and the monuments in Washington D.C. Crowd support was unbelievable. The water and food stops were well-stocked and well-organized. This race is also extremely popular. Registration had filled in just 23 hours, so I was thankful to be there.

The 10K course starts at the Mall and follows the last six miles of the marathon. The marathon itself starts at the Pentagon and finishes at the Iwo Jima Memorial.

Cheryl Monnat joined me on the trip and was going to run the 10K race. We stayed in the D.C. suburb of Arlington and decided not to rent a car. The D.C. metro system is clean, safe, and efficient, so it was easy getting around all weekend. Our hotel was only a half block from the metro station.

We had also chosen our hotel because it was the closest one to the finish line. Being close to the finish line is a real plus when you have to walk back to the hotel after the race.

Once we arrived in DC, our first task was to go to the Marine Armory to pick up our race packets. All the pick-up points were stationed by Marines. Pick-up and everything else associated with the race were models of efficiency, fast and glitch-free. Trust the military to have everything running like clockwork.

Cheryl and I flew in on Friday to give us some time to relax before the Sunday race. On Saturday, that part of the East Coast got a surprise early snow storm. So instead of sightseeing, we went to the local movie theater near the hotel to catch a movie. It is always a good idea to stay off your feet as much as possible the day before a marathon.

That evening, we had the pleasure of having dinner with Ruth and Richard Cook, two Team CMT members from Virginia. I had contacted them a few weeks before the event to see if we could meet. Most people with CMT don't know anyone affected by CMT outside of their family. Richard has CMT and is a also a marathon runner. Athletes with CMT, especially long-distance runners are rare, so it was great to meet and share experiences with this special couple. We felt like we were long-time friends.

Dinner was at a sports bar where the University of West Virginia was playing on every TV in the place. Every time the Mountaineers scored, all the fans would sing the John Denver song, *Take me home, country roads.* I guess it is a school tradition. Every time I hear that song, I am going to think of Ruth and Richard.

I had a great night's sleep (6 hours) thanks to prescription sleeping pills. With the exception of one other race, this was the only time I slept all night before a half or full marathon. Having a sleepless night before a marathon is probably pretty common among runners, but think about running 26 miles on little or no sleep. I had also been fighting a number of minor injuries in the weeks leading up to the race. I woke feeling energized and after breakfast, announced myself ready to go.

The morning was cold. It was only 34F. My feet and hands were numb from the chill for the first five miles. The race started with an osprey helicopter flyover, a prayer, and words of encouragement from comedian Drew Carey.

Carey has become a long-distance runner and ran the Marine Corps Marathon as his first marathon. He lost 60 pounds by running and has become a huge advocate for the sport. Drew fired the starting gun and we were off. Runners are seeded according to their start time. Because I would take almost five hours to complete the race, my wave was near the back of the 30,000 runners. The fastest runners start at the front, which is okay with me. I would not want to get in their way. Because I was seeded so far back, it took me nine minutes to get to the starting line. When we crossed the Potomac River to run into D.C., I could see the runners stretched out for miles.

I decided to just have fun with this run since I had already qualified for Boston. I took a small disposable camera with me to take pictures along the route. It was the most fun I have ever had running a marathon.

The crowd support was incredible. Marines manned all the water stops and in many spots, cheered us on along the course. At the Lincoln Memorial, we ran through a tunnel of people, the road so narrowed by the crowds that there was only room for only a couple of runners on the course. People cheered, "Go Team CMT!" Tears fill my eyes just remembering those voices floating through the crisp fall air.

I did get a little tired at mile 23 and walked for a mile, but felt good and finished in 4:57, four hours and fifty-seven minutes, ahead of lots of racers.

Later, Cheryl, running the 10K, told me she had had a rough start. The bridge over the Potomac River was icy and at least one runner fell. Cheryl finished in a little over 57 minutes—a really nice run—just one week after another half-marathon and about a month after her finish at Lakefront Marathon in Wisconsin.

For me, the best part of the whole day was getting my finisher medal. A Marine places the medal around the neck of each finisher. If you ever want to participate in a well-run, "big time" race, think about running the Marine Corps Marathon. It will be an experience I will carry with me for a lifetime.

After receiving my finisher medal, I met up with Cheryl and we went to get our belongings. Every runner checks the things they do not want to carry on the course at a baggage check. This marathon had the most efficient system for checking and retrieving luggage I had ever seen. Luggage pick-up was easy since we had been assigned a numbered UPS truck and a slot in each truck corresponded to your race number. This was typical of the outstanding logistics of the entire event.

I felt really good after the race. My legs were sore, but I really wanted to get out and see some of the city.

The Martin Luther King monument had been along the course, but I did not remember seeing it, so Cheryl and I went back to have a look. To get into town, we had to take the subway. I wore my Team CMT jacket. A number of people asked about it and I got to help them understand Team CMT and raise some awareness.

Cheryl and I walked around the mall a bit and then celebrated with dinner. We spent the day after the marathon touring the Capitol, the Supreme Court Building, and the Library of Congress.

Throughout our sightseeing, we saw several other marathon finishers. If you go to a event with a big out-of-town presence, you can tell the runners the next day. They are all pretty stiff and sore. Some were wearing Marine Corps shirts, others you could spot just by the way they were walking, especially stairs. Going down stairs the day after a marathon is even more painful than going up right after a marathon due to lactic acid build-up in the muscles.

Later in the day, we took a flight back to Milwaukee... a successful trip with another marathon of Boston qualifying time.

Chapter 17
Boston Marathon Application

*A man must love a thing very much if he not only
practices it without hope of any fame or money,
but even practices it without any hope of doing it well.*
—G.K. Chesterton, British author and journalist

This quote can certainly apply to my running. I am no longer very competitive due to the CMT, but I keep running and competing anyway. For all its challenges, running and competing bring me great joy. I feel good for hours after a good run or bike ride. I live to measure myself in a race. I love the day-to-day challenge of completing a marathon training program. But these "runner's highs" pale in comparison to being able to achieve a long-held goal.

For years, I have dreamed of running in the Boston Marathon, the Super Bowl of running and yardstick for any runner. A Boston Marathon jacket is a coveted item.

The week after the Marine Corps Marathon, I sent the Boston Athletic Association a letter to apply for entry in the 2012 race. I asked Joyce Kelly to help me because she is an author and a fellow Team CMT member. Joyce was able to talk with B.A.A. officials and helped to educate them on CMT. She really helped to pave the way. Many thanks to Team CMT member Joyce Kelly for helping me put this letter together:

RE: Boston Marathon 2012, Mobility Impaired Division

Dear Registrar:

My name is Chris Wodke and I am applying for admission to the 2012 Boston Marathon in the Mobility Impaired Division. I am a 53-year-old female runner with Charcot Marie Tooth Disease (CMT).

CMT is the most commonly inherited neurological disorder affecting 150,000 Americans, but most people including most medical professionals have never heard of it. I am raising awareness of this insidious disease by recently organizing Team CMT, a group of 21 athletes in 8 states.

Running the Boston Marathon is a major component of my mission to raise awareness of CMT. In addition to competing in as many running and triathlon events as we possibly can, I established a web site and blog where I raise funds and awareness of CMT. You can learn more about this irreversible condition at the site; www.run4cmt.com

CMT causes progressive deterioration of the feet and lower leg muscles, resulting in foot drop, tripping, falls and fractures. Additionally, it causes muscle tightness in the calves and constant burning and tingling in the feet as the nerves die and the muscles atrophy. It also causes these identical symptoms in the arms and hands.

For me, CMT means blisters and burning when I run and declining run times as my leg and foot muscles weaken and atrophy. I do not have enough flexibility in my legs to walk properly, much less run. Additionally, CMT causes profound fatigue. The rigors of marathon training are a day to day challenge. My doctors are amazed I am running any distance, much less distances of 26.2 miles. It is unheard of in a patient with CMT. Despite the CMT, I have completed five marathons including the Madison Marathon this past May, with a finishing time of 4:51. Moreover, the Madison Marathon is a very hilly course. Due to CMT, regardless of how much I train, I cannot achieve the normal qualifying time standard.

With this letter, I am supplying the following documentation for my mobility impairment:

- *Letter from local MDA office. CMT is one of 40 neuromuscular diseases covered by MDA.*

- *Diagnosis by Dr. Linn of the MDA Clinic at Froedert Hospital in Milwaukee*

- *Physician's notes from Dr. Lobeck with initial diagnosis of Type 1a CMT.*

- *Letter from the CMTA documenting CMT limitations regarding mobility*

Please let me know if there is anything else I need to supply or what additional steps are necessary to apply for the 2012 Boston Marathon. Acceptance to this race will be an important step in making the public and health professionals aware of this disorder.

Recently, I was told by two physical therapists people with CMT cannot run. I have 4 athletes on Team CMT suffering with this condition. We want to show the world our love of running and competition and we will not be stopped by CMT. Through participating in various running competitions, together we will strive to achieve our dream of a "World without CMT." Raising awareness is the first step on that journey.

I know there are many worthy athletes hoping for a bib in the Boston Marathon.

I respectfully request you give my application serious consideration. I am not running for myself, but for the 150,000 Americans with CMT, for my family members with CMT and for the other members of Team CMT with this disease.

Thank you very much for your time today. I sincerely look forward to hearing from you soon.

Very truly yours,

* * * * *

In re-reading this letter, I realize how much Team CMT has grown. We were really new then, back in 2010. As I am writing this book, we have grown to more than 100 members and have had 26 athletes affected by CMT on the team at one time or another.

* * * * *

Learning the proper application process for the Boston Marathon was my biggest hurdle. It took a few phone calls to get all the information. If accepted, I would pay my entry fee of $110 like any other runner and receive all the benefits of any entrant in the field.

Thousands of runners train and run, hoping for time to qualify them for this race. Then when registration opens, they apply with thousands of other hopefuls.

Like them, I would have to wait. When I left Milwaukee for the Marine Corps Marathon at the end of October, I had still not received a decision. I had made repeated phone calls to clarify my status. Hotels fill up quickly for the event and since it takes months to train, I would need to start training soon.

In addition, soon after I applied, I discovered that not everyone was supportive of my decision to apply to run in the Mobility Impaired Division of the Boston Marathon.

Chapter 18
Am I a Scammer?

We will go to the moon and do other things,
NOT because they are easy but because they are hard.
—President John F. Kennedy

After the registration for the 2011 Marathon filled in less than eight hours, in 2012, Boston Marathon organizers changed their registration process. Now runners are registered on a rolling basis, starting with runners having qualifying times less than 20 minutes from the time standard. As a Mobility Impaired runner, I was allowed to register at any time while the process was open. I had already submitted my letter and medical documentation to the Boston Athletic Association, the B.A.A.

I set running Boston as a goal, not because running a marathon is easy, but because it is hard. Boston is one of the toughest races to get into and one of the toughest to run. I am running it because many in the medical community think those with CMT can't run. I am running to raise awareness about CMT and to educate the public about those of us with this debilitating disease. I want those with CMT to know that it's possible to accomplish many things even with this disease. I am running to blaze a trail for my other team members with CMT.

I quickly learned that the B.A.A. had been clueless about CMT. In the future, when a Team CMT athlete applies to run Boston, the BAA will at least have heard of the disease.

Excited about getting closer to my goal, I shared with a co-worker about my Boston application. To my face, he told me I was a scammer. I was just like one of those people who is healthy and parks in the handicapped parking spaces. He said I was taking the place of someone who deserves to be there, like an amputee. When I explained that I have an inherited neuro-muscular disease, he stated that there was nothing wrong with me since I run marathons. He said it in such a matter-of-fact way, like there could be no other opinion about it.

His perspective bothered me, because I also wondered how I would feel lining up with other athletes who are ampu-tees or otherwise mobility-impaired. Of course, I don't want to take the spot of anyone who deserves to be there. The division is reserved for those athletes with conditions that prevent them making the time standard.

My CMT prevents me from making the standard no matter how hard I work. Boston is the place for top runners to compete. The fact that I am an hour under the time standard, even with CMT, shows I deserve to be there. Any of the other runners on my team with CMT would be hard pressed to make the 6-hour time standard. I came within 10 minutes of making the time standard years earlier and had CMT at that time.

It bothers me is that no one knows about CMT. If I had told my co-worker I had multiple sclerosis, MS, he would have nodded his head in recognition and that would have been the end of the conversation. In actuality, there are more people with

CMT than MS in the United States. While I can't do anything about CMT, I can at least do my utmost to make CMT a disease everyone has heard about.

Lots of people have conditions that aren't visible. Just because someone looks fine does not mean he or she is healthy. Many challenges people deal with every day are unseen, to be endured in silence, and even in shame. Conditions like lupus, depression, or MS are not visible but present challenges for those affected.

My co-worker's comment that nothing could be wrong with me because I run marathons hurt the most. Many of us with CMT look okay and the challenges we face are not visible to the average person. Even someone like me, with a mild case of CMT, faces challenges every day. Some days, I have profound fatigue, which makes it tough to get through the day, much less work out when I get home. I am much, much more vulnerable to injury than people without CMT. I can't run every day. My ankles don't have enough range of motion to walk properly, much less run. Researchers estimate that it takes a person with CMT twice the energy to do tasks like walk than the average person.

So not only am I a slower runner due to CMT, it probably takes me twice the energy. Imagine being out there running for five hours, expending twice the energy of the average runner. Just training for and completing a marathon with CMT is a major feat. In the back of my mind, I always have the message that this progressive disease might eventually steal my ability to run.

I am grateful for my co-worker's skepticism. His words made me even stronger in my conviction that I deserve to be at Boston and will line up proudly for Team CMT if the Boston Athletic Association accepts me.

I don't know if I will run in Boston next April. If I'm not accepted, it just means God has something else in mind for me. If that makes me a scammer, I am willing to live with that.

Chapter 19

Boston Marathon— Am I In or Out?

You can chase a dream
That seems so out of reach
And you know it might not ever come your way
Dream it anyways.
—Martina McBride, singer

From the first time I ever trained for a marathon, my goal was to run Boston. The closest I came to meeting the time standard was my first marathon. I ran it in four hours, missing the time standard by 10 minutes. As my CMT has progressed, that dream has gotten farther and farther away.

In mid-November 2011, my marathon dream became reality. I was informed by the Boston Athletic Association that I had been accepted to the Mobility Impaired Division. I had plenty of time to begin training and planning for Boston.

On April, 16, 2012, I will line up with 30,000 other runners and I will be representing Team CMT. I am going to get a medal. Every runner finishing Boston gets a finisher medal. The finisher medal from Boston is a prized procession for any runner. Medals are given to the top three age-group athletes, master athletes, and wheelchair participants. For most runners, the finisher medal is the only medal they ever get.

I am going to raise a lot of awareness and hopefully some money for CMT research. I am so proud and humbled to be running to raise awareness for everyone battling this disorder, especially those on the team with CMT.

While running Boston is a major goal, I have a bigger one: a cure for CMT. I want to have back what CMT has taken away. I want everyone I know who wears braces because of CMT to know what it is like to walk without them. I want everyone who struggles to do everyday tasks, like opening jars and buttoning buttons, to do them with ease. I know it seems like just another dream that's out of reach. I am going to dream it anyway. Not too long ago, Boston seemed out of reach for me, too. There is no end to what you can accomplish with a goal and a dream.

Excitement floods through me. I can't believe I will start my training in a month. It will be a tough road ahead, but I can't wait to get started. As the date of the race gets closer, fears and doubts and anxiety will come to the forefront, because I know how tough marathons are. Boston will be my seventh marathon. I know it will all be worth it.

Chapter 20
Boston Marathon Training Plan

Live a life worthy of your calling.
—Ephesians 4:1

My training for the Boston Marathon 2012 starts in December 2011. It takes 18 weeks to train for the event. I don't want to just run at Boston—I want to run well. I'm not running for myself anymore. I represent everyone on Team CMT, the HNF, and everyone struggling with CMT. I want to train hard, to respect the tremendous honor I've been given.

Running and raising awareness have become a calling for me. In April, 2012, I will have the chance to raise awareness of CMT on a huge stage. It is estimated as many as 500,000 spectators line the Boston course. A lot of people will hear about CMT for the first time. One of my friends with CMT told me this week: "We're all counting on you." This is a hope I keenly feel and will work hard to fulfill.

So how will I get ready for my race? Boston is a hilly course with the notorious Heartbreak Hill between mile 20 and 21. The first ten miles are downhill.

I've modified my training plan to account for the hills. That means lots of hill repeats. A hill repeat is exactly what it sounds like: running up and down hills again and again.

The training program for a marathon is 18 weeks long—four and a half months of committed effort. Consistency is the key to success. That means logging lots of miles during the winter. Sometimes I just won't feel like training. On some days, the weather just won't cooperate. Winters in Milwaukee mean months of cold, ice, and snow. Even on days when it is warm enough to run outside, high snow banks and icy sidewalks make running a chancy activity. So that means running on a treadmill to get in the requisite training.

I am a little apprehensive going into this training since I'm fighting injuries on both feet. This will be my third marathon in one year. That's a lot to ask of anyone, much less a runner with CMT. I have never trained for a marathon this early. Many of my workouts will happen in the cold and dark, so will need to choose between snowy, cold streets and the treadmill. I will have to balance training hard, but doing so in a way that will allow me to get to the starting line as healthy as possible.

Training for Boston is going to be a mental and physical challenge, one I gladly take on to fulfill my mission of raising funds and awareness for CMT.

Chapter 21
Week 1: Boston Training Race Against Time

The Finish Line isn't given, it's earned.
—Unknown

WEEK 1: DECEMBER 18, 2011
MONDAY—3 MILES EASY
TUESDAY—SPEED WORKOUT
WEDNESDAY—3 MILES EASY
THURSDAY—5 MILE TEMPO
FRIDAY—3 MILES EASY
SATURDAY—5 MILES MARATHON PACE
SUNDAY—10 MILES LONG, EASY

At our Team CMT debut race, I fell during the cool down period after the race. Before that, I had never fallen—before, during, or after a race—although I often fall or trip during training. That day, I had just seen an ex-boyfriend two years after a particularly nasty breakup. So maybe I was a bit distracted. You see, I have to concentrate on every step when I run. If I don't, a fall or stumble is likely.

An occasional stumble when my right foot catches is not unusual. Falls are nothing new, either, since skinned knees were a matter of course throughout my life. I always joke that even though I fall a lot, God gave me rubber bones.

Over the last year, my left foot has started to catch as well. My right foot has been catching and dropping for years. Foot drop, is one of the signs of CMT and is the inability to lift the front part of the foot. In general, foot drop stems from weakness or paralysis of the muscles that lift the foot, which causes the toes to drag along the ground while walking or running.

To avoid dragging the toes, people with foot drop may also lift their knees higher than normal. Or they may swing their leg in a wide arc. My legs swing from the hip when I run so that my foot can clear the ground. Most runners roll along their foot from heel to toe; I swing my legs around to clear the foot drop and then land. It works but it is kind of like having a break that stops me a little bit with every step. Sometimes, I don't clear completely and my foot catches, especially on my right side.

In addition, I have little flexibility in my legs and diminishing padding on my feet. Although I have the wonderful ability to point my toes, my feet don't bend so well in the direction needed to run.

The stumbles are even worse when I am tired. This week, I stumbled half a dozen times in the hours following my run. I had left on my running shoes and the thick soles might be more than my tired legs could handle.

I once asked one of my team members if he ever fell during a marathon. He said he usually falls several times during a race. I made a promise to myself if I ever start falling during races, I would quit competition. A fall could mean an injury and an injury could also end my ability to compete.

Injuries can happen at any time. Any rock, crack in the sidewalk, or uneven surface could mean an ankle roll or fall. I know a slip or trip at any time could have resulted in missed training, an injury, and possibly a missed race. Getting to the starting line healthy is a feat, especially for someone with CMT.

A fall could spell the end of training. One day, early in my training, I returned from the grocery store. It was snowy, so I piled my groceries in the hall leading to my kitchen. Going into the kitchen, my toe got caught on one of the bag handles. My toe stayed there, while the rest of my body lunged forward. I can still remember the pain of hitting the floor. Nothing severe, just bruising.

I have to pay attention to every step or risk a fall because I catch my foot. Walking is such a simple act and most of us never give it a thought. It is just part of our daily routine.

Only one percent of Americans have ever finished a marathon, so I'm part of that unique group of people with determination, stamina, and commitment to the marathoner's life. Every time I train for a marathon, I realize it could be my last. My CMT is progressing to the point where I may have no choice. If perseverance has anything to do with it, I will be in Boston.

* * * * *

Monday was day one of my 18-week training program for Boston. The week did not start well.

Sunday night, I only got about two hours of sleep. I tossed and turned most of the night and was still awake at 3:15 a.m. I was exhausted but my body just would not sleep even after two doses of Tylenol P.M. My legs were jumpy and I couldn't get comfortable. That happens to me fairly often, especially on Sunday nights.

I've struggled to get to sleep my entire life. It is one of the things that comes with the whole CMT package. There is no one set of symptoms that every person shows with CMT. Issues with sleep are one that can show up...lucky me.

Most mornings, I feel like I never slept and tiredness is my almost constant companion. Sometimes the fatigue is profound and I still have to go out and run or swim or do whatever is on the training plans. Other days, I feel really good and full of energy. I never know what each day will bring. I do know that each day no matter how I feel, I will tackle whatever challenges the day brings. If that means getting up and going to work on two hours sleep or doing a workout, I will get it done. I know that I really earn those finish lines.

* * * * *

Well, the alarm went off at 5:15 and I went through the mental struggle I go through every time I have a sleepless night. My body is telling me it needs sleep and to call in sick. My brain tells me I haven't called in sick in nine years and "You aren't starting now."

I was meeting a friend for dinner, so if no work, no dinner. The brain won. Imagine having to work all day, socialize, and come home and go through a workout on two hours of sleep. That was nothing compared to the five marathons I have run on no sleep. But starting the week exhausted is not helpful when trying to keep up with a marathon training program. That evening, I was able to get in a 45-minute workout on the Nordic Track and crashed at 8:30.

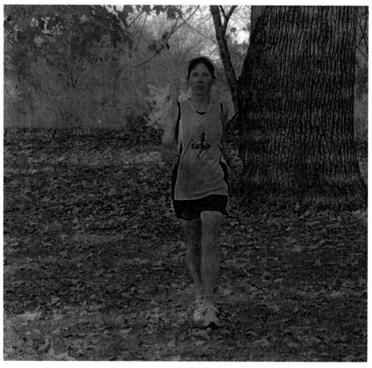

Fall is my favorite season for running.

Chapter 22
Team CMT Partners with HNF

Desire is the starting point of all achievement, not a hope,
not a wish, but a keen pulsating desire
which transcends everything.
—Napoleon Hill, author

Right before I got accepted to run Boston, I saw a Facebook posting about someone running the Richmond Marathon to raise money for CMT research. Of course, I posted a comment trying to recruit her to Team CMT. In the past, I'd used the Internet and Facebook quite a bit to find members for Team CMT. It turned out that the runner was the sister of Allison Moore, president of the Hereditary Neuropathy Foundation (HNF). Allison wanted to discuss a partnership with the Hereditary Neuropathy Foundation (HNF).

I gave her a call and we had instant rapport. We decided to meet in person to discuss a possible HNF sponsorship of Team CMT. To save some money, I would fly and stay with my sister in the Philadelphia area and Allison would drive down from New York to meet me.

Before Allison arrived, I met up with one of our local team members, Jude. I got to also meet Jude's adorable daughter, 14-month-old Harmony. Jude recently had run the

Philadelphia Half-marathon on November 20th as a fundraiser for CMT. So I got to hear about her race and share experiences of being an athlete with CMT. What a pleasure to meet Jude in person after seeing so many Facebook posts and exchanging emails. The best part about starting Team CMT has been meeting the other members. I never expected the team to grow so large or meet so many other athletes fighting CMT, with the same challenges and same athletic interests as my own.

Allison took a couple of wrong turns getting to my sister's house and was a bit late. We had the same rapport in person that we had over the phone. We talked about the team and she told me about some of the work HNF was doing and how Team CMT fit in HNF's mission.

One of the projects HNF sponsors at the University of West Virginia is studying the effect of exercise on CMT. HNF's sponsorship of this type of research showed a true understanding of the importance of exercise. Allison understood right away how Team CMT could help to raise awareness and funds for research. I could tell Allison had a great vision and Team CMT fit perfectly with HNF.

After discussions with Allison, I decided to affiliate Team CMT with the Hereditary Neuropathy Foundation (HNF.) This was not an easy decision, since, like many team members with CMT, I am a also member of the CMTA. I decided to partner with HNF for the following reasons:

- The foremost reason is the passion and vision Allison Moore brings to the table. Allison has CMT and at one point in her life, was training to run the New York Marathon. She understands the challenges being an athlete with CMT. Even more importantly, she is an enthusiastic supporter of our efforts. In talking to her, I realize our visions are closely aligned. I think Team CMT and the HNF are a perfect fit.

- The HNF is offering financial support for team uniforms and a website. To date, I had been funding the team out of my personal resources. HNF help will free up my funds for my training and contributions to CMT research. I also need additional help in managing this team. We have grown to 62 members and I expect we will grow even larger. We have grown so large that managing the team has become a part-time job. I feel if I need to turn over team management to HNF at some future date, the team would be in good hands.

- The HNF provides much greater exposure and visibility for our team. They have created a tab for Team CMT on the HNF website. They also use social media to promote the team; HNF will be posting my blog entries and tweeting updates using their social media. There may be a media day soon in New York for video for the HNF web site.

- HNF has greater media connections and visibility than I do. My mission in starting the team was to promote awareness of CMT. HNF will partner with us to get the story out about the amazing athletes on our team. This will be especially important as I run the Boston Marathon this year and other team members run Boston or other high- profile events in years to come.

- I support the HNF model of fundraising through athletic events and its support for physical activity by those with CMT. HNF's experience in doing fundraising will be helpful. There has already been talk about HNF helping to put together an event in Richmond next year. Hoping to get many Team CMT members to that event.

- My fundraising efforts in Boston will go to fund the research on the effect of exercise on CMT. This study is headed by Dr. Robert Chetlin at the University of West Virginia Medical School. This study is being done in partnership with HNF.

The only difference for the team that affiliating with HNF would be a new uniform. Getting the uniforms done this time was a much quicker process. Allison and I agreed to work together in early December. The first CMT/HNF shirts were ready for a half-marathon in Allen, Texas on December 31, 2011. I even had a hand in designing the new uniform. I remember seeing HNF's triad design on its website. I knew it would be perfect for Team CMT.

I still planned on being a member of the CMTA and continuing my fundraising efforts for that organization. I was grateful for CMTA's support and the use of the STAR logo on our current uniform. The move to affiliating with HNF was about being a sponsored athlete. I believed we were all in the same fight. We were all working toward the same cause, treatments, and a cure for CMT.

After a CMTA patient conference in Chicago late in 2012, which I did not attend, the CMT-affected English/American triathlete again posted negative comments about Team CMT on her blog. She stated that we were standing in the way of a cure and members should think twice about the impacts of wearing the Team CMT uniform. She had once been a member of Team CMT and was the only one who objected to the HNF partnership. She started posting negative comments on our Team CMT Facebook group. I removed the posts, which led her to post several negative things about me on her Facebook feeds. I "unfriended" her, for I did not want her opinions to negatively influence the team.

She asked to be removed from the team, which I welcomed. She had never been an active member or ever very supportive our cause. I think she felt we took the attention away from her. Until we came along, the CMTA thought she was the only athlete with CMT. So she was a shining star for them until I came along and our team stepped into the spotlight.

I believe the CMTA contacted several team members regarding the alliance of Team CMT with the HNF. Several Team CMT members quit, stating that they viewed CMTA as the only hope for a cure or because they did not like the negativity.

I did my best to keep things positive, privately sending the triathlete an email asking her to stop posting the negative comments in her blog. I told her I admired her commitment and passion for the CMTA and asked her to respect that I had equal fervor for my effort. I shared that I feel the effects of CMT every day since my dad is in a wheelchair and the cost to care for him is quite high due to that. Without my permission, she put the first few lines in the comment section praising her. I asked her to take it down since the email was selectively quoted. She did and then asked me never to contact her again, a request with which I gladly complied.

I don't like non-profit "wars." MS has five different groups raising funds and advocating for patients. I do not know why the CMTA thinks the CMT world is not big enough for both the HNF and the CMTA. We are in the same fight; we should be fighting CMT, not each other.

Chapter 23
Why Running?

*I believe God made me for a purpose.....But he also made me
fast, and when I run, I feel His pleasure.*
—Eric Liddell, from the movie *Chariots of Fire*

Wisconsin has long, cold, dark winters. Sometimes it seems like the sun does not shine for weeks. Running in winter means bundling up for sub-zero temperatures or navigating icy roads.

The weather presents a challenge. It's definitely hard to get out the door to run in the winter. The training program for Boston is 18 weeks long, meaning I am training all through the worst winter months in Milwaukee. Winter means cold, dark days and it gets dark at 5 p.m. We get lots of snow and cold. Many days the temperature is below zero. The sun warms the sidewalks during the day and then re-freezes as the sun goes down. So often the sidewalks I need to run on are icy. If I am really desperate to run outside, I will run in the street. The city salts the streets and the pavement is almost always dry and ice free. Sometimes I procrastinate for hours.

Spring is not much better. It seems to take forever for winter to give way to warmer weather. Summer is great and fall in Wisconsin is golden. Fall is my favorite time for running. The trees turn shades of red and gold, and brown leaves crunch under my feet as I run my favorite routes. The experience is so precious because the warm, sunny days are numbered.

On days like that, I know exactly how Eric Liddell felt. I had a 20-mile run to do today. As I went out the door I realized it was one of those days we all live for in Wisconsin. Fall is my favorite season and it was a perfect fall day. If I never ran again, I would want to remember this as my last run.

I ran on sidewalks colored gold with fallen leaves. Part of my run followed the Lake Michigan shore and the water matched the color of the sky, both sapphire blue. It was warm with just a slight breeze. What at day for a run and to be alive! There really is a runner's high and I am going to feel great for hours. Days like today are why I run.

I got to run through six parks along my route, all full of fall foliage of gold, red, and green, all lit by golden sunlight. I will carry the memory of this run through the long winter months ahead. I am not fast, but I felt the pleasure of being a runner and being alive on such a fantastic day.

I get the same pleasure out of biking, skiing, swimming, or whatever physical activity I do. Long before I was a triathlete, I used swimming and biking as cross-training. Running every day is hard for most athletes, and my CMT-affected body cannot hold up to the daily pounding. So I run every other day and do pool running, biking, skiing swimming on the days when I don't run. They are all part of my training routine.

I love the feeling of the wind in my face when I ride my bike. It's the same joy and freedom I felt when I was a kid riding around the neighborhood with my brothers.

Skiing gets me outside during the winter in Wisconsin. It gives me something to do and keeps me from getting cabin fever. I am both a Nordic (cross-country) and an Alpine (downhill) skier.

Nordic and Alpine skiing are really opposite experiences. Alpine is speed and the wind in your face. It took me a long time to master downhill skiing. I now revel in every turn because it has become second nature. I have been a member of the National Ski Patrol for 25 years.

Nordic, or cross-country, skiing is more of a quiet pleasure. Gliding along in the woods is peaceful and contemplative for me. Usually I am the only person on the trail. I love the peace and quiet among the beauty of trees covered in snow. I don't get out nearly as often as I would like. I fall quite a bit when I cross-country ski and worry about getting injured. I am so used to shifting my weight and using my ski edges to turn with downhill skis; my cross-country skis do not have edges.

Kayaking and hiking provide more opportunities to be outdoors. Wisconsin has lots of great lakes and hiking trails. Some of my best memories are kayaking in Northern Wisconsin in the Land O' Lakes area. I often visit in the fall. By and large, the tourists stop coming after Labor Day. I have paddled the Manitowish River in the fall. I remember paddling on sapphire-blue water, the banks lined with trees shimmering in the breeze with golden leaves and I had it all to myself. Just me and the wildlife I saw that day. Kayaking on a day like that feeds my soul.

I feel so alive and am so keenly aware of the pleasures running, biking, and my other outdoor activities bring me. I hope I am able to enjoy them all for many years to come. There is no guarantee with CMT, so I treasure each experience and every good day I have.

When I told my friend Kathy about my CMT and my plans to run Boston, she also asked me "Why running?" I keep running because I am trying to save a part of who I am. Maybe I should not define myself by being an athlete. My athleticism is hard won and I'm not ready to give it up yet. I know that running and being active are my best shot for leading a fulfilling and normal life.

Someday I my CMT may force me to stop running, but for now, I am going to use being active, especially running, to keep me strong and slow the progression of my CMT.

Chapter 24

Week 2: Boston Training
My New Running Partner

The secret to success is persistence.
If one way doesn't work then try another.
—Unknown

WEEK 2 –DECEMBER 25, 2011
MONDAY—3 MILES EASY
TUESDAY—SPEED WORKOUT
WEDNESDAY—3 MILES EASY
THURSDAY—5 MILES TEMPO
FRIDAY—3 MILES EASY
SATURDAY—5 MILES MARATHON PACE
SUNDAY— 11 MILES LONG EASY

I arrived in Dallas during the middle of Week One of training for Boston to spend the holidays with my brother Tony, sister-in-law Cindy, and my nephews Brandon and Dan. The winter weather in Dallas is almost always better than we have in Wisconsin. This trip was no exception. Temps were in the mid 50s to upper 60s. It wouldn't be the weather's fault if I didn't stick to the training plan.

I had a long run of ten miles scheduled for Christmas Day and had entered a half-marathon race on New Year's Eve morning. I also had two five-mile tempo runs to do. Tempo runs are an even bigger challenge than just running and I often put off doing them. I also wanted to do some speed work, plus figure out what to do for exercise on the days I didn't run. Tempo runs are part of the speed work runners do to get faster and stronger. To do a tempo run, I warm up for ten minutes then run at my current 10K race pace, followed by a ten minute cool down.

Fitting in runs around all the holiday prep and family time can be really tough. Christmas day, after we opened presents, everyone else in the house was napping and I was really tempted to skip the run. In addition, I sometimes felt guilty slipping out for a run when I could be visiting with my family. Sometimes I heard, "You're exercising again?" although on this visit, everyone knew I had a marathon to get ready for in April. My motivation needed a little nudge and I got just the energy boost I needed from my nephew Dan's dog, Mojo.

Dan is a business student at Texas Tech, majoring in accounting. He and Mojo were home for the holidays. Mojo is a chocolate Labrador/Australian Shepherd mix and at a little over a year old. He still has his puppy zest for life and his company was just the assist I needed, especially since I am training without any music. I planned on running the Boston Marathon without my iPod, mainly because it has become a distraction.

Mojo was my running and walking companion for all but one day of my visit. Seeing how much he enjoyed going for a walk or run really got me out the door. The only day we missed was the day I ran the half-marathon in Allen, Texas. No dogs were allowed or I might have considered taking Mojo. He literally pulled me along when walking and I had a hard time keeping up when running. He has an endless source of energy.

It was fun to have Mojo join me for my runs and walks. He really loves to be outdoors and his excitement was infectious. It helped me to remember the joy of running and just being outside.

Running with an overgrown puppy is a bit of a challenge. He had his own agenda when we were together and often stopped dead in his tracks to check out something of interest. Sudden changes in direction happened often as well. We also seemed to find where every dog in the neighborhood lived, since they greeted us with growls and barks.

One dog threw himself against the fence as we passed. That scared Mojo into the street, taking me with him. When I looked back, I saw what looked like a Doberman jumping higher than fence height to get a peek at us.

Thanks, Dan, for letting me train with Mojo. I'll miss him. I was able to get in every scheduled running workout, though missed a weight lifting session or two. Mojo seemed to take my attempts at weight lifting as an opportunity to play.

The half-marathon went well and I am pretty healthy. I am right on track for Boston so far.

Chapter 25
My Most Memorable Christmas Gift

Success is not final, failure is not fatal.
It is the courage to continue that counts.
—Winston Churchill, British Prime Minister

As I was getting ready for Christmas with my family in Texas, I thought about the gifts I've gotten through the years. My most memorable Christmas present was a pair of ice skates I received when I was ten years old.

My parents never had a lot of money and with seven kids, buying Christmas gifts must have been a challenge. Most years, we had piles of presents under the tree. I think most of the year, my dad worked two jobs, not only to pay Christmas but for all the other expenses of raising a big family.

That year, my mom told me I could only ask for one present, so I gave that gift long and hard thought. My older brother is learning disabled, and the school system was not offering much help, so my parents were getting him support on their own, which strained the family budget. My parents just could not afford more than one gift per child. Money was so tight, there was not even money for a Christmas tree. I remember, though—we had two trees that year; we just did not pay for them. My dad sort of waited for the lot to close on Christmas Eve and obtained two for us.

On Christmas morning, the most beautiful pair of ladies figure skates was waiting for me. Even though it was the only gift I got that year, I learned a few things from the experience.

Focus: When you have to whittle down your list to one gift, you focus on the one thing you really want and you had better make it count. It takes that same kind of single-mindedness to be successful as an athlete. Whether it's running for a cure for CMT, entry into the Boston Marathon, or working on a swim stroke—focus is the key to success. I figure out what is most important to me and set my goal.

Visualization: I remember watching Peggy Fleming skate and I wanted to do that, which is why I asked for skates for my one present. The day after Christmas, we were going to my grandma's house on Okauchee Lake, about thirty miles west of Milwaukee. I knew I would get to try out my new skates. As I lay in bed that night, I visualized every part of how it would feel to skate. Well, the realty was a little harsher than my child's picture.

With my CMT-weakened ankles, I could not stand on the skates, much less glide across the ice. But that skill of picturing success has stayed with me throughout my athletic career.

Determination: Although my first skating attempts on the frozen Wisconsin lake were a disaster, I kept at it. Any type of sport for someone with CMT requires lots of hard work. It takes the muscles longer to learn and retain a skill than a normal athlete.

Running has made my ankles strong enough to be able to skate. It is just as good as I imagined all those years ago. While I won't be doing any spins like Peggy Fleming, I can make it a whole hour without falling. Funny that I should remember that single gift from over forty years ago and what it taught me with such clarity. I was not sad to only be getting one gift, just grateful and appreciative for the present I received. I made the most of it. I learned it is challenge that changes you and you learn more from mistakes than success.

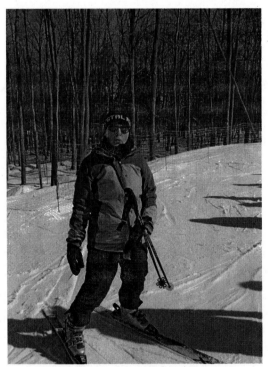

Later my love of skating turned to skiing.

Chapter 26
Week 3: Boston Training
I knew I Could Run a Marathon When.....

At mile 20, I thought I was dead, At mile 22, I wished I was dead. At mile 24, I knew I was dead. At mile 26.2 I realized I had become too tough to kill.
—Unknown

WEEK 3— JANUARY 1, 2012
MONDAY—3 MILES EASY
TUESDAY—SPEED WORKOUT
WEDNESDAY— 3 MILES EASY
THURSDAY—4 MILES TEMPO
FRIDAY—3 MILES EASY
SATURDAY—6 MILES EASY
SUNDAY—8 MILES LONG EASY

I never grew up thinking I would run long distance. I remember running relay races in grade school and being screamed at for being slow. Plus my knees were perpetually skinned from falls (all due to the CMT). Not a good start to a running career.

I was never athletic but had always been active. I played tag, football, and baseball with my brothers. We rode our bikes everywhere and as long as I didn't compare myself to anyone else, I enjoyed being active. I started running in college to become a better skier, an activity I still do every winter as a member of the Crystal Ridge Ski Patrol in Franklin, Wisconsin . It was like that with skiing. I got up and fell down a lot, but I mastered skiing and have been a member of the National Ski patrol for over 25 years.

I started racing after college. I used to tag along to races with Cheryl Monnat, a sorority sister from college at the University of Wisconsin–Milwaukee. I never remember winning anything and being really slow, but it was fun. We went often, even competing in a 10K at Badger State Games.

The first time I won a medal was at a 5K race as part of a conference. It was a really, really small race. I won my age group three years in a row and was hooked. I became friends with a local running coach and talked him into training me. He taught me how to do speed work and tempo runs. I would often place in my age group and even won the women's division of a 2-mile race once. For the first time in my life, I felt like an athlete.

One day, as part of my long run, my coach asked me to run for an hour without my headphones. He said it was important as a runner that I listen to my body. I did it and liked it. I loved paying attention to my body and everything happening around me instead of just listening to music. It made me feel strong

Music had become such a crutch for me. I did not think I could run without it. If I could run for an hour without music, I could run a marathon.

I completed my first marathon in four hours and I did it without headphones. Finishing that marathon made me feel like I could accomplish anything. I've done five more and I have that same feeling of accomplishment every time. I know I'll get that same feeling again when I cross the finish line at Boston in April.

Finishing marathons has carried over into my whole life. When I set a goal, I know I am going to reach it, whether it's running Boston, a project at work, or raising money for CMT. Most goals are a lot easier than running a marathon without music.

My third week of training for Boston was also the week that Team CMT and the HNF formally announced their partnership.

I had already run the Denton Half-marathon in Texas on New Year's Eve wearing the new Team CMT-HNF singlet. Here was the press release for the big announcement!

Team CMT and the Hereditary Neuropathy Foundation join strides in the race for a cure!

Two organizations of like mind and motivation unite to create an even greater impact. Team CMT, a force of 62 and counting, are athletes dedicated to raising awareness of Charcot-Marie-Tooth, the most common hereditary neuropathy that results in loss of peripheral nerve functioning and muscle atrophy. And yes, many of team members themselves have CMT! The Hereditary Neuropathy Foundation (HNF) is a non-profit organization dedicated to raising CMT awareness and funding research into treatments and a cure.

HNF was founded by Allison Moore, who was training for a marathon herself when an increase in her CMT symptoms sidelined her just before the New York marathon in 2001. Since then she has dedicated her life to supporting those with the disease and finding a cure.

I was very excited about the partnership. What I did not expect was the reaction I would get from many in the CMT community.

Chapter 27
A New Uniform for Team CMT

*After climbing a great hill, one only finds
that there are many more hills to climb.*
—Nelson Mandela

Team CMT and HNF also unveiled the new uniform
design (shown opposite). This logo made its debut at
the half-marathon on December 31, 2011 in Allen,
Texas. The athletes of our team will be wearing this logo as we
complete in triathlons, walks, bike rides, runs, and spin events.
Members will wear this logo as we raise awareness of Charcot-
Marie-Tooth Disorder, or CMT.

Team CMT is comprised of 62 athletes from 16 states
united to find treatments and a cure for the condition that
affects 155,000 Americans. CMT is the most common inherited
neurological disorder.

Team CMT is now sponsored by the Hereditary Neuropathy Foundation. The HNF was founded by Allison Moore when
she got a sudden onset of CMT symptoms from cancer
treatment. She, like the other members of Team CMT, is
dedicated to raising awareness of CMT and helping those
affected to live healthy and active lives. HNF is very active in
raising research through athletic events, so there is
great synergy!

Lots of thought and discussion went into the design. The three triangles represent the three universities partnering with HNF to do research: University of California—Davis, University of California—Los Angeles, and University of West Virginia School of Medicine. This is part of the TRIAD logo. TRIAD stands for Therapeutic Research in Accelerated Development.

The concentric circles in the middle of the green triangle represent a Schwann cell. The Schwann cell is a cell of the peripheral nervous system that wraps around a nerve fiber and forms the myelin sheath, which is needed for speedy nerve conduction. In CMT 1a, which is the most common type, the ability of Schwann cells to maintain the myelin sheath is impeded by overproduction of a protein.

You can also see the figures representing the sports in which Team CMT members are active. Typically the swim would be represented first since swim, bike, and run is the competition order for triathletes, but the majority of our team members are runners and walkers, so we left the runner at the peak. The two websites are also on the logo to promote our team and to educate about CMT.

I will be running wearing this singlet in the Boston Marathon this April. In addition, I will be raising money to fund research of Team CMT athletes by Dr. Robert Chetlin at the University of West Virginia School of Medicine. He will be studying the CMT-affected athletes on the team to measure the effect of exercise on the cells and nerve sheath. Those of us on the team with CMT already know how beneficial exercise has had been in our lives. We have seen progression slowed and in some cases reversed with running and other vigorous exercise. Dr. Chetlin's work will aim at recommending appropriate exercise for CMT patients.

It is an exciting time for our team. The new uniforms are to be sent out at the end January. The whole process of coming on board with the HNF went really smoothly. It took months just to get a logo for our shirts from the CMTA. We are looking forward to adding many new members. I expect we will reach my goal of 100 members well before our one-year anniversary at the end of April, 2012.

Little did I know the uproar that our partnership would cause within the CMT community.

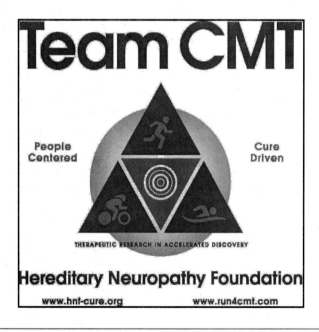

Chapter 28
iPod Banned in Boston

*Success is to be measured not so much by the position
one has reached in life as by the obstacles
he has overcome while choosing to succeed.*
—Booker T. Washington

The Boston Athletic Association strongly suggests
runners not listen to music while running the Boston
Marathon. There isn't an outright ban except for those
competing for prize money. My ban is self-imposed. I will not
be wearing my ipod in Boston; in fact I have stopped using it
for workouts and other races as well. For a lot of reasons it just
seems like the right thing for me to do:

It's Boston
The most important reason is to honor the race. The Boston
Marathon is the oldest and most prestigious marathon in the
world. It is a tremendous honor to even be running. I am one of
a limited number of runners accepted into the Mobility
Impaired division. We're in the very first wave to take off, even
before the elite athletes. I just don't feel like I can line up in
that group wearing headphones.

Pioneering

The first woman to run in Boston was Katherine Switzer in 1967. Officials tried to pull her off the course. She finished the race and many women have followed in her brave footsteps. Now 53 percent of marathon fields are women. When Katherine ran, it was thought long-distance running was harmful to women and they should not run anything longer than a 10K. We athletes with CMT hear something very similar. We are told not to do anything too vigorous and many of us have been told running is harmful. I may be the first athlete with CMT to run Boston, but I won't be the last. Team CMT has three other members with Boston qualifying times. I am going to show just how strong those of us with CMT can be and hopefully lead the way for many more Team CMT members to run Boston. I don't want to do anything that would make B.A.A. officials think twice about having CMT affected athletes run.

Mental Toughness

I want to run the best possible race I can in Boston. I ran my first two marathons without music and have not completely run one since I started using music. I think I need to be just a bit tougher mentally to complete the Boston course without walking. It takes lots of stamina and determination to finish a marathon, especially on a hilly course like Boston. I am going to need every bit of mental strength. I've already stopped wearing my iPod to train and race. I actually really enjoying listening to the world around me.

Scoring

Walking means a longer finishing time. Because the Mobility Impaired division has about two dozen athletes, I have a chance to medal. I don't want to blow that chance by walking. Because this may be the only time I run Boston, I want to have the fastest time I possibly can.

Focus

I want to concentrate on how my body is feeling. I want to experience the sights and sounds without a sound track. Sometimes a song or the volume on my iPod causes me to lose focus. Going without my iPod means one less thing to worry about on race day.

The focus helps me to have better workouts as well. The lack of music helps me stay in tune with how my body is feeling. This is very important for effective workouts and preventing injury. Plus I get great ideas on my runs that I just don't get when I listen to music.

Safety

Some of my workouts have been outside after dark. Running in the dark with headphones is really a bad combination for safety. I am always leery about running after dark, but have had to several times this winter. Being able to hear traffic and other things around me is very important for safety.

Team CMT

I'm not running for myself anymore. I represent a team and we're sponsored by the Hereditary Neuropathy Foundation. By the time Boston rolls around, we may have additional sponsors. I want to represent my team and sponsors well. To me, that means looking like a serious athlete. You won't see an elite athlete wearing an iPod. Plus quite a few people are coming out to cheer me as I run the course. I won't hear them with music playing.

Vanity

Earbuds sticking in my ears just look bad. I don't feel like I look like an athlete. I've worked so hard to achieve this goal and I want to look good for all the photographers along the course; I plan on buying lots of pictures. It's totally vain; I admit it. Working on a great wardrobe for Boston as well. If you can't be good, you have to at least look good. That Team CMT singlet will look terrific at Boston.

Triathlons

I started competing in triathlons shortly after I was diagnosed with CMT. Headphones are not allowed in any portion of the triathlon, so it was a good idea to get used to training and competing without them.

I don't want to criticize anyone wearing headphones. There have actually been some studies that show listening to music can increase performance. If it's the thing that gets you out the door to exercise, that's good as well. I used music for years and sometimes it helped get me moving.

Now, music has become a distraction. I want to run a race worthy of my calling to raise awareness and funds for CMT research. Running without music is the right decision for me.

Chapter 29

Week 4: Boston Training
Working Hard

If people knew how hard I worked,
they wouldn't be so amazed.
—Michelangelo

WEEK 4: JANUARY 8, 2012
MONDAY 3 MILES EASY
TUESDAY SPEED
WEDNESDAY 3 MILES EASY
THURSDAY 6 MILE TEMPO
FRIDAY 3 MILES EASY
SATURDAY 7 MILES MARATHON PACE
SUNDAY 13 MILES LONG EASY 13

In Wisconsin, if you don't like the weather, just wait a while. Week 4 training brought a couple of challenges, not the least of which was the weather. It was 57F when I left work on Wednesday afternoon. The day before, it had been in the low 50s and I managed to get in a bike ride for my training.

I got my speed workout and tempo run in on Monday and Wednesday when the weather was still nice. A tempo run is where you warm up for a mile, then run at about a 10K pace for all but the last mile, which is run slowly to cool down. Intervals are usually run on a track. I've gotten hurt twice running on tracks, so I just run for time. I take my 5K pace and estimate the time it will take me to run whatever is on the plan. 5K pace is the speed you would run in a 5K race, or 3.1 miles. In the beginning, the intervals are 200 meters. As the weeks go on, the intervals run will get longer and more varied. By the end, the intervals are multiples of a mile.

Thursday we were hit with six inches of snow and much colder weather. I did the Nordic track on Thursday and a pool run on Sunday. A pool run is just what it sounds like. My health club pool is shallow, only chest deep. I run back and forth in one of the lanes just like I would outside. I started running in the pool when I got a stress fracture training for my first marathon. I discovered I could not run every day so I run outside or on the treadmill on one day and run in the pool on other days. I get one or two more days a week running by running in the pool.

Saturday came around and the morning temperature was 16F. That was just too much of a change to do an outdoor run. Plus there was too much snow and ice. I just couldn't risk a slip or fall.

So it was off to the gym for a 13-miler on the treadmill. Based on my latest half-marathon time, I knew that would take 2 hour and 45 minutes. It takes some determination to grind out such a long treadmill workout. Having the TV helps, although there is not much worth watching on Saturday morning. I was able to get some hill work in, so it was nevertheless a good workout.

Treadmill workouts were a matter of course when I trained for the Madison Marathon last year. We got 22 inches of snow on Groundhog Day. The snow banks at the corners were so high I was worried about a fall if I ran outside. All that climbing also gets in the way when doing speed work and tempo runs.

In addition, with my mom in the hospital, the treadmill was sometimes the only way to get in a workout. My work gym was just a few blocks from the hospital so I could see her, go get a workout, and return to the hospital if needed. I was able to get in every workout, only missing the day she passed. I am nothing if not determined. Too bad I don't have the talent to go with the drive. That would really be a combination.

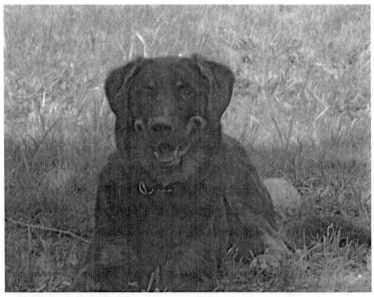

My favorite running partner, Mojo.

Chapter 30
I'm Still a Scammer

If you do good, people will accuse you of selfish ulterior
motives. Do good anyway.
—Kent Keith, author of *The Paradoxical Commandments.*

I saw the co-worker who had called me a scammer. I asked him if he had checked out the Team CMT website. He said he had and yes, he still considered me a scammer. He said I run marathons so there is nothing wrong with me. I did not say much. He is an engineer and engineers always think they are right. I know because I am an engineer and am a little bit that way myself. Well, as a rule, they're pretty smart people and because of that, there is no use responding to a statement like my friend made. There is not much point in arguing. It is just a waste of time.

I think of my CMT as like a house with termites. A house with termites looks fine, too. You would never guess there is a problem deep inside. With CMT, my nerves are being attacked just like the wood in a termite-infested house. I feel a little frustrated for being so successful in working to overcome my CMT.

My co-worker made an assumption that because I look fine, I must be fine. If he would have asked some questions and been open to learning, he might have learned a bit about what it is like to live with CMT.

Having CMT means my body does not regulate temperature well. I am almost always cold. I keep my electric blanket on my bed all year round. My hands and feet are often like ice. I have to wear chemical warmers on my hands and feet when I do my ski patrol shift and still get cold. I have to take a warm bath when I get home or I shiver for hours, even under an electric blanket and down quilt.

Having CMT also means I am tired all the time. It is estimated it takes twice as much energy for a person with CMT to do daily tasks. This is due to the breakdown of the nerves. As already mentioned, I have had trouble falling asleep my entire life. Sometimes I am awake all night. So imagine coming home to do a 9-mile run and being so tired, you just want to sleep. Imagine doing a marathon with little sleep and the energy that has to be expended to complete a race that takes five hours.

One of the symptoms of CMT is very, very tight calf muscles. I have little flexibility in my ankles. This means my feet don't have the flexibility to walk correctly, much less run. Plus the tight muscles set me up for injury. It is really tough to get in the training needed to be successful without getting injured.

I have scoliosis, a curve in my spine, which is also common in CMT. My hip is also rotated up and to one side on my right side, so sometimes it really feels like one leg is shorter when I run. I have a great chiropractor who is working on this and does his best to catch any injuries early.

The worst thing about the CMT is the progressive muscle weakness. Because the nerve signals slow, the leg and arm muscles slowly die. Any layoff for injury or an accident can see acceleration in weakness. It may be just a matter of time that I will be so slow it will not make sense to compete. It is tough to watch my skills go more quickly than others my age. The muscle weakness causes foot drop. So my foot catches causing me to trip, especially when I am tired. So I have to pay attention every time I run and even more so after a race.

CMT affects my hands as well. I am losing some of the fine motor control to do things like type.

I'm not complaining. I know I am so, so lucky to be running, especially in a race like the Boston Marathon. So many people with CMT wear braces and have problems doing simple things like opening a jar or buttoning buttons. My CMT is considered very mild and although I run marathons and look fine, I still have challenges.

I certainly don't expect anyone to throw a parade in my honor. I'm no superhero. I am just an ordinary person with goals and a lot of drive. I never expected to be accused of having selfish motives.

We all have lots of work to do to educate people about living with CMT. I know I've seen enormous benefits from exercise. Some of my symptoms have even gotten better.

I hope most people will be inspired by the athletes of Team CMT. At the time of my conversation with my friend and co-worker, there were sixteen athletes on the team with CMT. They bike, do triathlons, and like me, run marathons. Like me, they have drive and a love of being active.

So call us scammers if you will, but take the time to find out what a person with CMT goes through each day before you judge.

Chapter 31
Week 5: Boston Training
The Glamorous Life of an Athlete

We all have dreams. But in order to make dreams come into realty, it takes an awful lot of determination, dedication, self-discipline, and effort.
—Jesse Owens

WEEK 5: JANUARY15, 2012
MONDAY—3 MILES EASY
TUESDAY—SPEED WORKOUT
WEDNESDAY—3 MILES EASY
THURSDAY—7 MILES TEMPO
FRIDAY—3 MILES EASY
SATURDAY—7 MILES MARATHON PACE
SUNDAY—16 MILES LONG EASY

Fatigue starts to be a problem at this point in the training. My body handles any stress by sleeping. Stress from work, a cold, or tough workouts all are dealt with by sleeping. Both the workouts and work have been tough this last week. Plus the CMT brings fatigue.

About 75 percent of those with CMT report problems with being tired. Sometimes I am so tired, I want to go home and go to sleep, but have to work out. Sometimes it's tough to talk myself into working out. Of all the things I face from the

CMT, being tired all the time is the worst. Being tired takes a mental toll as well. It is so difficult to wake up tired each day. It is so hard to get through a work day when I have gone three or four nights without a good night of sleep. At least once a week I have a night where I struggle most of the night to fall asleep. Imagine after struggling to get through the day due to fatigue or a sleepless night and having to come home and do a workout. The good thing is I usually feel a bit better both mentally and physically after working out.

Saturday, I had a ski patrol shift at Crystal Ridge, a local ski hill. Some nights at the hill, it's cold or the runs are icy, so lodge sitting and socializing rather than skiing are more the norm for the guests. But that night, the snow was good, and I got in lots of ski runs.

Sunday I had a 16-mile treadmill workout. It took 2 hours and 54 minutes. I threw in 1 hour and 20 minutes of hills as I begin to train for the Boston course.

Sunday night I was exhausted from the weekend's activities and in bed at 6 p.m. I fell asleep reading about 6:30. I pretty much slept through until 4 a.m. the next day. Fatigue haunted me the rest of the week, though. Monday, all I wanted to do was go home and go to bed, but I had a speed workout to do. So it was out the door for a 50-minute speed workout. I'll be in bed by 8 p.m. That's living in the fast lane, all right. I can't remember the last time I've been to a party or happy hour.

The weather was up and down all week as well. Monday was 41F and by Wednesday it was 6F. So it was back to the treadmill again for both my tempo and long runs.

The treadmill is hard on my feet. As the CMT progresses, I am losing the padding in the bottom of my feet. I'm told that is a normal part of the progression. Sometimes I can really feel the pounding. I have been fighting a turf toe issue on my right toe since last summer. It is an overuse injury from all the running. The area right at the base of the big toe gets really sore. You don't realize how much you use a body part until it gets injured. The big toe is critical for balance in running and walking. As the foot rolls during the running stride, the area at the base of the toe bends to push off. So it is not a good injury to have. It is still tender and I used tape for my long run.

My other big effort this week has been fundraising. Saturday I spent all day emailing potential corporate sponsors. I think I sent close to 60 requests for funding. I am getting about a 10 percent response to fill out applications.

The training is going well other than the tiredness. This week is an easy week. The training plan builds for two weeks then cuts back on mileage for a week before ramping up again. It is a much-needed physical and mental break.

This week ends with a 10K race with Team CMT team members Cheryl Monnat, Robert Kearney, and Kathy Stultz. We will be racing in Franklin, Wisconsin, as part of the Racers Against Childhood Cancer winter series and then going to the Great Lakes Multi-Sport Expo after the race. I am hoping to look at a triathlon suit and maybe some bikes at the expo. It is also a great place to scout out runs and triathlons for the upcoming season.

Chapter 32
Challenges are Opportunities

Opportunity is missed by most people because it is dressed in overalls and looks like work.
—Thomas A. Edison

Last night, Milwaukee Brewer's Centerfielder Ryan Braun accepted his MVP award from the Baseball Writers of America. Braun. At the time, most valuable player and Milwaukee hero, now is serving a 50-game suspension for alleged steroid use.

"Sometimes in life we all deal with challenges we never expected to endure," Braun said. "We have an opportunity to look at those challenges and either view them as obstacles or as opportunities, and I've chosen to view every challenge I've ever faced as an opportunity. And this will be no different....

"I've always believed that a person's character is revealed through the way he or she deals with those moments of adversity. I've always loved and had so much respect for the game of baseball. Everything I've done in my career has been done with that respect and appreciation in mind, and that's why I'm so grateful and humbled to accept this award tonight."

How Braun addresses the fans on his return and how he deals with the issue of his steroid use will be a true test of his character. As an athlete, I have always admired I hope I will be proud of how he faces the challenges before him.

I think back to my own challenge when I was diagnosed with CMT in 2010. I recognized the tremendous gift I had because I was able to still run. I feel blessed because my CMT is mild and my symptoms have allowed me to stay active. I saw my ability to run long distance as a tremendous opportunity to raise awareness of CMT. I chose to celebrate the fact I can still run and will seize the opportunity to make the most of it. I know every workout and every race brings us one step closer to raising awareness and a cure. I realize life will bring challenges both good and bad. I can't choose what happens to me, but I can choose how I react. My life will be defined by the choices I make and how I choose to walk—or in my case run— the path set before me.

John Ortberg said in his book, *The Me I Want to Be*, "Rising to a challenge reveals abilities hidden within you and beyond you that would have otherwise remained dormant" and "When adversity comes, you find out what you are really made of."

I see these truths every day with the awesome athletes on Team CMT. When I founded the team, I never expected to find other athletes who share this disease. I've been told by many medical professionals that people with CMT can't or shouldn't run. I never expected to run the Boston Marathon, yet in April, I will be at the starting line. Team CMT has three other runners with Boston qualifying times and I hope to see them on the starting line next year as well. Each month we seem to add more CMT-affected athletes to the team. At the time of the writing of this book, we have over two dozen.

We have athletes preparing for the Ironman in Florida, as well as the National Triathlon Championships. The members of this team are determined not to let their CMT define them and to enjoy the sports they love. As they battle the effects on CMT on their athletic abilities, they point to a hope beyond themselves, because they run, play football, ride, spin, and tri for everyone else affected by CMT. We know we are so blessed when so many with this disease wear braces to walk and struggle with everyday tasks like writing, fastening buttons, and other tasks of daily living.

So thanks to the athletes on the Team with CMT and thanks to their family members and friends who support us by being on the team. All of us realize CMT may one day take the ability to enjoy the sports we love. Until then, we will work to raise awareness of CMT and face our challenges with the same grace and optimism that has marked our efforts since our inception.

So, thanks to the members of Team CMT. You are an inspiration to me and to the entire CMT community!

Chapter 33

Week 6: Boston Training Racing

Only those who risk going too far,
can possibly find out how far they can go.
—T.S. Elliot

WEEK 6 – JANUARY 22, 2012
MONDAY—3 MILES EASY
TUESDAY—3 X HILL, 1 DOWN
WEDNESDAY—3 MILES EASY
THURSDAY—5 MILES TEMPO
FRIDAY—REST
SATURDAY—6 MILES MARATHON PACE
SUNDAY—1 HOUR 20 MINUTE RUN

Week 6 was one of my easy weeks of training. Every three weeks, I cut back the mileage to give my body a chance to rest and recharge. I needed it. Instead of a long run this week, the training plan called for a 10K race and I joined Team CMT members at the RACC Winter Series 10K Expo Run.

It was a snowy and windy day. The race organizers did a good job of clearing off the bike path. The starting temp was around 27F, but the brisk wind made it feel much colder. We started off into that wind. I asked team member Cheryl Monnat after the race if she ever has thoughts about turning back in a race or bailing at the half-way point. I know I did for a brief time. She said she did that day, which made me feel a bit better. Last year, the course was two loops. The 5K runners did one loop and the 10K runners, me included, did two. It was tough to see them all finishing and know I had to run the same course all over again. This run also has a wooden bridge about a mile into the course that runners need to cross twice, or four times for the two loops. With all the runners going across, that bridge really bounces and it feels pretty weird if you aren't in sync, which I wasn't. It was actually a bit unnerving.

All in all, the race was a good way to end my rest week I ran the race at an easy pace to use it as a training run, finishing right around 1 hour. I am never happy with my time. It is always slower than I want. I used to be able to do this distance in about 48 minutes. Now due to the CMT, I am much slower. Every race reminds me.

I got to talk with teammate Kathy before the race. She and her son Lincoln run for Regan, her daughter and his sister. Lincoln was away for his high school ROTC team. I missed him. It is really wonderful to see a brother running for his sister and experience that kind of family support. Kathy' and Lincoln's efforts remind me why I started this team and why I am running the Boston Marathon this April. We always run for those with CMT who can't, like Regan.

After the run, we went through the expo and checked out clothes, potential races, and lots of fancy bikes. I saw a wonderful Trek Madone 5.9 racing bike I would love to have. Gotta start saving for that.

Even though it was an easy week, I was exhausted by Sunday night and again in bed by 6:30. Sometimes the CMT really wipes me out.

Back to the hard training next week. I have an 8-mile tempo run, an 18-mile long run, speed work, and an hour and a half pool run this week. That is in addition to cross-training, weightlifting, and ski patrol duty on Saturday night. I'll take Monday as my one rest day this week because honestly, I'm too exhausted to work out. No excuses the rest of the week.

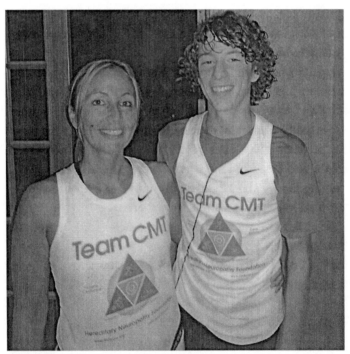

Kathy and Lincoln Stultz, proud members of Team CMT

Chapter 34

A Small Piece of the Wall

*No one could make a greater mistake than he did nothing
because he could only do a little.*
—Edmund Burke

B urke might have been talking about a Jew from ancient
times named Nehemiah. Before Christ was born, the
Jews were conquered and the wall around their city of
Jerusalem was left in ruins. They were forced to leave
Jerusalem and marched to Persia.

An ordinary Jewish man, Nehemiah, was the cupbearer to
the King of Persia. This ordinary man had a vision to return to
Jerusalem to rebuild the walls and protect his people. He had a
vision and the courage to approach the King to make it happen.
He asked for safe passage, permission to rebuild the walls, and
materials to do it. He took the risk and it paid off.

When he arrived in Jerusalem, he assigned each family a
small portion of the wall to rebuild. After lying in ruins for 95
years, the walls were re-built in 52 days. The build wasn't easy;
the Jews faced ridicule and opposition from their enemies.
People in the country surrounding the city tried to keep the wall
from being rebuilt.

But they got it done and fulfilled this leader's vision. The
Jews were able to return from exile and defend Jerusalem. His

efforts helped prepare the way for the return of the Jews to their city.

This story comes to mind as I have also experienced opposition from members of other CMT-related organizations. Many in the CMT community saw Team CMT's joining HNF as some kind of betrayal. They try to tear down the work we do. Many of them are not doing any work to raise funds or awareness, but they are willing to try and dare down my efforts and those of my team. Raising awareness is laying the foundation for finding treatments and a cure.

Raising money is another essential step in the effort to raise awareness. People give money because they know someone with CMT. Raising CMT awareness is my vision and my small part of the wall. Having athletes wear our Team CMT jersey may seem like a small piece, but every seemingly minor act may have influence beyond our knowledge.

Many in the CMT community seem to content to sit on the sidelines. They don't get involved in fundraising, donating to the efforts of others, or even raising awareness, yet they are willing to criticize the efforts and post negative comments of those on Team CMT who are making a contribution.

For instance, when the trailer for the film *Bernadette— Living With CMT* was released, several members of various Facebook groups who are neither affiliated with HNF nor CMTA began posting negative comments on Facebook about how the subject of the movie must be making lots of money from it. The woman in the documentary, released in 2010, is severely affected by CMT. She lets a camera follow her along as she goes to doctors and physical therapy appointments and lives her life. She made no money off of the project. So instead of posting negative comments, it would be nice if some of those people took some time to consider what part they might play to help find treatments and a cure.

Like those families in Jerusalem, Team CMT members continue to work on our small part of the wall. Every race we run, every dollar we raise, every story published, every radio and TV interview, is just one more piece of the wall.

Our hope is a world without CMT. I can do only a little, but am proud to be even a small part. I hope others will join us. We welcome anyone to join us in this fight.

Chapter 35

Week 7: Training for Boston
What a Difference a Year Makes

No matter how bad you feel, there is always someone
out there who feels worse and is still moving.
—Popular runners' saying

WEEK 7: JANUARY 29, 2010
MONDAY—4 MILES EASY
TUESDAY—4 X 800, 400
WEDNESDAY— 4 MILES EASY
THURSDAY—8 MILES TEMPO
FRIDAY— REST
SATURDAY—7 MILES MARATHON PACE
SUNDAY—16 MILES LONG EASY

Saturday was a perfect day for my long run. It was 39F and I had a gorgeous run along the lake and even did over an hour of hill work by running up and down a couple of hills on the route.

Last year on Groundhog Day, which fell during this week, we got 22 inches of snow. We got so much snow and it was so windy that my back door was drifted shut. The snow was so deep, I had to put on snowshoes to get to get my shovel out of the garage. It took me six hours to dig out. After I was done digging out, I went running. It's really fun to run in the snow.

The challenge came after the storm, when every street had snow banks three or more feet high. It got to the point I was worried about getting hurt climbing up and down the banks every block. Plus the sidewalks got really icy from the freezing and thawing and salt. Most of last February, I spent using the treadmill.

Saturday's long run was somewhere between 16 and 18 miles. My goal was to run for 3 hours and 6 minutes, planning for 18 miles based on my last half-marathon time. I tried wearing a GPS watch last year. It is supposed to measure distance based on satellite reads, but was wildly off so I gave up on it and resold it on Amazon.

I don't seem to have very good luck with watches. It doesn't matter how expensive they are, they never seem to last long on my wrist. They simply stop working. My latest watch casualty was one I inherited from my mom. It lasted about four days before it stopped working. I have no idea why I have such bad luck with watches. Do I put out bad energy? Do I have bad body chemistry? No idea. My running watch is the only one that seems to work consistently.

The training plan called for 16 miles, but I am trying to extend each of my long runs by a couple of miles, hoping that will make me a bit stronger so I can hold my pace throughout the marathon.

The toughest part of the long run is getting out the door. Whether I think of the long run as the 18 miles I want to do or the 3 hours and 6 minutes I knew it would take—it just sounds really far. It can be tough to get motivated to get started. I had some letters to mail, so the first step was running to the post office and then to just keep going. My plan was to find a hill or two and do repeats. Repeats are just as fun as they sound. I run up and down the hill again and again. It trains my body to run hills. Since Boston is a hilly course I need the practice. I ended up down along Lake Michigan and had a great run. I was in bed by 6 p.m. both Sunday and Monday. In fact, Monday I was so tired, I couldn't work out. The week's rest day got moved from Friday to Monday, which allowed me to get in all my other workouts, including an 8-mile tempo run. It is no big deal to miss a workout or two over the course of the training program. The key for me is to get in the three runs I need to do every week and move around the off-day as needed.

I also have a TV interview with the one of the sportscasters from a local TV station. The reporter is also doing the Boston Marathon, so she is interested in my story.

It is hard for me to believe the changes since last year. A year ago, I was training for the Madison Marathon, not knowing if I could even run a marathon again. A year ago, I was having trouble getting media attention. Now I have a publicist and several interviews pending.

A year ago, Team CMT was just in the idea stage. I had no idea we would grow so fast, that there would be so many athletes with CMT, and so many others interested in helping with our cause. What a difference a year has made.

I think amazing things are going to happen over the next year. I hope it is as good as this year has been.

It is also supposed to continue to be warm and dry this week. All good news for me as I continue getting ready for Boston!

Chapter 36
Fueled by Caffeine & Sugar

Running is a big question mark that's there each and every day.
It asks you 'Are you going to be a wimp or are
you going to be strong today?'"
—Unknown

Well, today I was strong, but I really wanted to be a wimp. I had a job interview today and a media interview yesterday so it's been a busy and important week. Last night, I woke up at midnight and it was hours before I was back asleep. So I started the day tired and went through two grueling hours with a panel of four interviewers, which added stress to being tired. Plus the interview was during lunch so my whole schedule was off.

On the training plan today is an 8-mile tempo run. I was really supposed to run that yesterday, but had to work late to make up for the time I took from work to do the TV interview. By the time I got home, the sun was setting. The thought of doing my workout in the cold and dark was a true turn-off. I was really, really tired, but tomorrow the wind chill is supposed to be 0F, so it has to be today.

It is always a juggling act for any athlete to balance a work and personal life against a training schedule. It gets more complicated with CMT, because I never know if I will get a good night's sleep or if I will feel too tired to work out. Sometimes I have to resort to desperate measures.

So I fueled up with a Pepsi. I told myself that if I didn't feel better, I could always do a treadmill workout tomorrow. That caffeine, sugar, and the prospect of a treadmill workout were just enough to get me out the door. Being successful as an athlete takes discipline and consistency, and sometimes the key is the mental tricks I have to use to keep me working out on my worst days.

I don't drink very much soda so Pepsi is a pretty good stimulant. I try to eat healthy so drinking soda to fuel a workout is not my normal routine. Sometimes I have to make a compromise to get the workouts done. Sometimes I have to work out no matter how tired I feel. All kinds of tricks with diet, moving workouts, and mind games come into play. For me, the training for a marathon is as much mental as physical.

Tempo runs are always the toughest for me. They start with a warm-up of ten minutes of easy running and end with ten minutes of easy running to cool down. Between start-up and cool-down are six miles at a 10K race pace for six miles, or a bit over an hour. My tempo runs were both mentally and physically challenging, because I was also including hills.

I won't lie—the tempo run was tough. I was tired and I did the same hill over and over, as hills are considered a substitute for a tempo run. I ran in the park just across the street from my house, so keeping the workout close made it mentally easier.

Plus I kept telling myself I am going to be really tired as I near the end of the Boston Marathon. So running when I'm really tired is both good mental and physical training for the end of the race. This is one workout I will store away in my good memories. I was not a wimp today. I made my 8-mile goal or 1 hour and 18 minutes. I feel good about overcoming the mental and physical challenges I had in getting out the door this afternoon.

Running strong and finishing workouts like these will make me strong both for my Boston race and all the workouts I have to do until then....even on days when I am really, really tired.

Chapter 37
CMT is our Mountain

The test we must set for ourselves is not to march alone, but to march in such a way that others wish to join us.
—Hubert Humphrey

Shortly after Team CMT partnered with HNF, I got a call from the President of the Charcot Marie Tooth Association, CMTA, in December of 2011. The association had shown no interest in the team until I started talking with the HNF. By the time CMTA contacted me, I had already agreed to the partnership.

Support from the CMTA included the use of their STAR (Strategy To Accelerate Research) logo and a couple of articles in their monthly newsletter. Before joining Team CMT, one of our members had contacted the CMTA to start a team. She was told "No, because people with CMT can't run."

Now that we moved to HNF, there was suddenly eager interest in us. My phone and email buzzed with messages from the CMTA to stay with them. Did they really want us or just to keep the HNF from having us?

One of the things I found frustrating about the CMTA is that it has pinned all its hopes on a drug cure for CMT. CMTA has been promising for some time that a cure is three to five years away. No drugs are currently being tested and it takes on average over ten years to get government approval for a new drug. Who is it kidding?

What if there are bad side effects? What if it so expensive no one can afford it? The HNF is funding drug research, but it is also funding research on the effectiveness of exercise on CMT. Any drug therapy may be more effective when coupled with exercise. But most people do not want to hear about exercise. The medical community used to tell people with CMT not to exercise.

Another thing that bothered me about the CMTA is it often seemed to feature cute kids in wheelchairs or other severely affected adults in its newsletter. Only about one percent of those afflicted by CMT end up in wheelchairs, but I guess cute kids bring in money—money needed for the large salaries of CMTA leadership. Only rarely did CMTA feature those overcoming their condition.

A merger of the two groups had recently fallen through and the relationship between the two was not good.

A few weeks after our press release about Team CMT joining forces with HNF, the CMTA started its own team, called CMT Athletes. Dee (not her real name), the former reluctant Team CMT member was one of the prime movers in starting the new team. A friend of hers designed the new team logo. She also posted several negative posts on our team site on Facebook. She did not really want to be part of our team, but had no problem starting her own. I think she perhaps missed being the center of attention when the CMTA thought she was the only CMT-affected athlete.

Here is the story I posted on my blog in response:

CMT is Our Mountain

Tenzig Norgay was a member of the first team to reach the summit of Mount Everest. He said about climbing mountains; "When people are going to a mountain they should forget the mole hills. When they are involved in a big thing, they should have big hearts to go with it."

He and Edmund Hilary were the first to me reach the top of Everest in 1953. No one knew if it was even possible, because many had tried and failed. After their feat, reporters wanted to know "Who got there first?"

Tenzing later wrote about the question: "Mountaineers realize there is no sense in such a question... two men are on the same rope, and that is all there is to it." He further said "All the way up and all the way down, we helped each other and were helped by each other and that was way it should be." He explained. "We were not leader and led, we were partners."

Those of us in the fight against CMT are partners as well and in a sense, on the same rope. All through my training, I have been helped by many of you with advice and encouragement. Many of us with CMT know it takes a big heart to do what we do and I could not run Boston without the support and encouragement of my team. CMT is the mountain we climb together.

As of today, there is a second group to raise awareness of CMT. The CMTA has decided to start a team. Some in the CMT community have been upset Team CMT is sponsored by HNF. We had at one time been loosely affiliated to the CMTA.

I am a CMTA member. I support its mission and wish this new team well. If I see the athletes at an event I will cheer them on and salute them as I pass them on the race course. I'll be happy to take a picture with them and even sign an autograph or two. Just kidding.

I refuse to engage in battle with them. I personally have spent over $10,000 dollars to raise awareness of CMT. I have CMT and have seen the effects in my own family and in the families of team members. The athletes on this team understand that CMT steals a piece of us every day. I am committed with my heart and soul to this cause. I am committed to each and every member of this team.

I welcome anyone wishing to climb this mountain with us. We are in the same battle and we are on the same rope. It doesn't matter who gets there first, who raises the most money or has the biggest team. I'm in competition against CMT, not another team with the same goal. When we find treatments or a cure for CMT we'll all be winners.

I am thankful for each of the members of this team. You all mean so much to me. I value each and every one of you. It means more than I can say, especially as I prepare for Boston.

Thank you so much for your encouragement, interest and support of Team CMT and our mission to raise awareness of Charcot-Marie-Tooth Disorder."

* * * * *

Shortly after the announcement of CMT Athletes, the CMTA Chicago Support group withdrew my invitation to speak at their meeting. The CMTA president lives in Chicago. Several people left Team CMT. I suspect they had been contacted by someone affiliated with the new CMTA team. Everyone who left had the same reason: they felt the CMTA was the only hope for finding a cure. Funny, I was told something similar by the CMTA president and the same words sometimes appear in CMTA literature. The HNF funds research at three universities and many programs to support patients affected by CMT.

CMTA members seem to think the HNF is in competition with the CMTA. The thought seems to be that the HNF takes scarce dollars away from the CMTA. Some members forget the HNF also funds research and has patient programs.

Never once have HNF personnel made a disparaging remark about the CMTA. I wish I could say the CMTA or some of its members had been as supportive.

I had planned to continue fundraising for both groups. After receiving the negative comments and emails, I asked the CMTA to take down my fundraising page. I was doing what I felt was best for the team and this cause. Who were they to criticize and try to pull the team apart? I was very disappointed and hurt by CMTA's reaction.

I still get negative comments from CMTA members in Facebook groups. It divides the community and does not help our cause. The world is most definitely big enough for both of us.

Chapter 38

Week 8: Training for Boston
Achieving Dreams

It's a dream until you write it down. Then it's a goal.
—Unknown

WEEK 8: FEBRUARY 5, 2012
MONDAY—4 MILES EASY
TUESDAY—4 X HILL, 1 DOWN
WEDNESDAY—4 MILES EASY
THURSDAY—6 MILES EASY
FRIDAY— REST
SATURDAY—7 MILES EASY
SUNDAY—12 MILES LONG EASY

Boston is 62 days away. That sounds so close. Last year, I wrote the date April 16th, 2012 on a piece of paper and put it on my bulletin board. April 16th is the day of the Boston Marathon. I don't remember the exact day I put up that goal, but I know it was soon after I was diagnosed with CMT. I put up that goal even before I ran my qualifying marathon in Madison. Somehow I knew I was going to be there. It is hard to believe my goal is so close. I've now replaced that goal on my board with my Boston acceptance letter.

I achieved another goal of sorts this week when I sat down for a TV interview with Trenni Kusnierek of WTMJ TV. I chose to run the Boston Marathon because as a high-profile event, I knew it would garner interest to raise awareness of CMT. I am not really an attention seeker. I am not the life of the party. However, I was willing to do media to raise visibility for our cause.

I have to admit I was a bit nervous before the interview. It was my first ever TV interview. Trenni put me at ease right away. She is running Boston for the second time and had some great advice to share with me.

For both of us, it will be marathon number seven. It was so much fun to talk about training and races with her. Thanks to my publicist Gail Sideman for arranging the interview. I also gave Trenni a Team CMT singlet and she promised to wear it. I hope to see her when I run Boston.

During the interview, Trenni shared that she had hurt her Achilles tendon and had not been able to run for three weeks. She is back to running so I wish her well and a good run at Boston.

Once the camera came on, I feel like I lost all ability to speak rationally. Pros like Trenni really earn their money. Thanks, Trenni and Gail, for helping me to bring awareness about CMT and the activities of Team CMT!

* * * * *

It is really easy to over-train when getting ready for a marathon. I am especially vulnerable to injury because of my CMT. I walk a fine line always between training enough to prepare and over-training and being injured.

At week 8, I am getting into the meat of the training program. I had a couple of nights this week when I woke up at midnight and couldn't fall back asleep, so finishing all the training this week was a challenge. I got in my speed work and 8-mile tempo run before it snowed and turned nasty cold. On Saturday morning, it was 8F with wind chills of -5F, so it was off to the treadmill.

At the gym, I did 3 hours and 24 minutes with hill repeats the entire time to simulate the hilly course at Boston. The steepest segments felt really good. My heart was going and I was breathing a bit hard. I loved the challenge of the hill work and it made the time go by fast. That 3-hour plus treadmill session was about the same as an 18-mile run.

I did a ski patrol shift on Saturday night and Sunday I was only a little sore.

Training is still going well. I have some tenderness around my right knee. I always have a bit of a problem with the muscle just left and below the right knee cap. It just needs stretching and some Bio-freeze®. I have trained for enough marathons that I know how to adjust my training and take of small problems as they pop up. Twice monthly visits to my sports medicine chiropractor, Dr. Drweiz, also keep me healthy.

This week is going to seem easy since it is a rest week. The number of miles build for two weeks and then cut back on the third week to give my body a chance to recover. This week, I have a race 10K race with Team CMT members Kathy Stultz, Robert Kearney, and Cheryl Monnat. I also have a speed workout and a long run of 12 miles. After my treadmill session, 12 miles sound easy.

Chapter 39

I'm Not a Scammer Anymore

Don't let what you cannot do interfere with what you can do.
—Coach John Wooden

I posted the on-line version of my article by *Journal Sentinel* reporter Tom Held on my cubicle bulletin board. The guy who had called me a scammer deems it my "I love me" board. I used to keep my finisher medals and numbers there until I moved them to my home office. Now the only things on the board are the article and the piece of paper with the Boston Marathon date.

The "scammer" guy walked by my cubicle and the article caught his eye, so he stopped to read it. I pointed out he was the one the reporter mentioned who had called me a scammer. Called me a scammer twice actually.

My colleague read the article and said he doesn't think I'm a scammer anymore now that he has been educated. He even said he was going to make a donation. The power of the media to change hearts and minds—amazing! I hope the media exposure has the same effect many times over.

He continued to read the article and noticed my goal time for Boston was 4 hours and 41 minutes. He asked me if I couldn't run faster than that, since that was only a 10-minute mile. I told him I would race him and though he might be faster, I could outlast him and explained that I was indeed running as fast as I could.

With the CMT, I told him, I'm also getting progressively slower. I can't run the marathon pace I used to run when I could run a 4-hour marathon. It's hard to watch others my age run the times I used to be able to run. I have to concentrate *not* what I have lost to CMT, but what I still have and what I can still do.

So I'm not a scammer anymore, maybe just a slacker for only running 26.2 miles at a 10-minute pace.

* * * * *

The power of the media is really amazing. Two of my co-workers approached me after the interview aired. One told me about her Lupus and the other about her Crohn's disease. Both women shared struggles they had with having an invisible condition. I am glad my being open about my condition helped them open up about theirs. It created a bond between us and we often discuss how we are doing with staying active.

How many others out there look just fine, but carry secret burdens? Some have Lupus, some have elderly parents or sick children to care for. So many people struggle with things we know nothing about. My heart goes out to each and every one of them. Sometimes we have no ideas what the truth really is.

Well, I have no control over the effect of the media or what anyone else thinks. I let them have their opinion and don't worry about it. It's really freeing not to be the slave of anyone else's opinion. I do what I think is right and let all the rest go.

I'm not going to get tied in knots because thinks I'm a scammer or a slacker or even if they think I'm some kind of hero. A few stories or TV interviews do not mean I am anything special.

Chapter 40
Week 9: Training for Boston
A Week of Ups & Downs

Running is the greatest metaphor for life
because you get out of it what you put into it.
—Oprah Winfrey

WEEK 9: FEBRUARY 12, 2012
MONDAY—4 MILES EASY
TUESDAY—5 X 800, 400
WEDNESDAY— 4 MILES EASY
THURSDAY—8 MILES TEMPO
FRIDAY—REST
SATURDAY—7 MILES MARATHON PACE
SUNDAY—12 MILES LONG EASY

To be successful as an athlete, you have to be consistent in your training. That means working out even when life throws you a few curve balls, even when you don't feel like it. This week definitely had its ups and downs.

My boss is retiring and a few weeks ago, I applied for her training manager position. On Monday, the hiring manager pulled me aside to tell me I wasn't even going to get an interview.

I've spent the last twelve years of my professional life getting ready to take this position. To not even get an interview was really devastating. I can honestly say I have still not completely recovered. I did not expect to get the job, but at least anticipated having a shot at it. I'm not sure what the future will look like in my professional life or what will happen next. I am certain there will be some significant changes sometime soon.

Honestly, some days it was tough to run, but I did get through the week. Saturday was the high point because five Team CMT members, including me, raced at the RACC Big Chill 10K in Pewaukee on February 11. Racing felt good after a tough week. This time, Kathy and her son Lincoln raced together. Lincoln is in 4th place in the points series for his age group of 14 and under. He did not want to wear his new singlet yet because he is waiting for his mom to customize the back with "Linco is a running fool."

The day did not start well for me because I had a fall in the parking lot. Leave it to me to find the one icy patch in the whole place.

It was a sunny and relatively warm 28F day. Cheryl Monnat took 2nd in her age group 50-54, just 20 seconds behind the winner. Lincoln medaled and I took 6th in my age group. My hamstrings hurt the whole race. Team member Robert completed the entire race on an injured heel. Kathy finished right alongside Lincoln.

I was too sore to do my long run on Sunday, so I did a run of 2 hours and 10 minutes in the pool. I occasionally have to substitute a pool workout when fighting an injury. It's OK, as long as it doesn't happen too often. Considering the week I had, I'll take it.

Chapter 41
Too Tired to Ride

There is a difference between interest and commitment.
When you're interested in doing something,
you do it only when circumstances permit. When you're
committed to something, you accept no excuses, only results.
—Art Turock, author and speaker on elite performance

The workouts aren't going to be any easier this week. On the plan are a 9-mile tempo run, some speed work, and a long run of 20 miles. Hopefully the rest of my life is a little calmer than last week.

If I buy a new bike, will I be too tired to ride it? That was the question I asked myself.

I attended the Multi-Sport Expo in January. My teammate Cheryl found some great deal on bike clothes. While I was waiting for her to checkout, I had the one of the salesman bring a Trek Madone 5.9 off of the rack. Just to look at, mind you.

The frame was a small so it was a pretty good fit. It had a gorgeous silver and blue paint job and although it was not the woman's specific model, it fit pretty well. The women's model was a not-so-sharp pastel mint green.

This bike has electronic shifting and a carbon frame. I could lift it with one finger. The price tag is anything but light, coming in at around $5,300. I am looking to upgrade my road bike, because to be competitive in triathlons, I need a better bike. The bike portion is the longest part of the race and a good bike can make a huge difference.

After I finish the Boston Marathon, I plan on doing the RACC duathlon series and several triathlons. I will also be attempting to qualify as a para-triathlete for the national championships. Still trying to figure out what races and how the process all works.

Sometimes I wonder if I am worth the investment in such an expensive bike. I wonder if I am a good enough athlete to justify the expense of a fancy new bike and I wonder if I will be able to use it.

* * * * *

On Sunday night, even though I went to bed early, it was after 3 a.m. before I fell asleep. The alarm went off at 5 a.m. I was so exhausted on Monday after work I couldn't work out, and was in bed again at 6 p.m. It finally took a prescription sleeping pill to get some rest. The prescription pill is one I resort to only when I am really desperate, since this type can be habit-forming. I wish I could tell you I woke up feeling well rested.

It is hard to explain how my tired is different from the tiredness everyone else feels.

When we had storms in Milwaukee, I often had to stay up all night at work as part of my job as a supervisor in the Control Center for a utility company. That kind of stay-up-all-night tired is how I feel when I have one of these days. I call it profound tiredness. It feels like I need to lie down and go to sleep and my body aches. Being exhausted takes an emotional toll as well. I was so low emotionally on Monday night I was in tears as I struggled to sleep.

* * * * *

When I get this tired, I wonder if this is the future I can look forward to. As my CMT progresses, will I be too tired to ride my bike or run or do the other things I love to do?

Right now, I am still able to work out most days, even on the days I am really, really tired. So will I get a new bike? Probably. Will it be a Trek Madone 5.9? Probably not, but I will get something to help me reach my next goal and continue to battle the CMT to be the best athlete I can be.

Will I be too tired to ride it? The answer will be yes, some days....but there are still more good days than bad days. I will cherish those good days and fight though the not-so-good days. That for me is what it means to be an athlete.

Chapter 42

Week 10: Training for Boston Running Your Own Race

We will win and live with it if we can't, but you will never know how far you can go unless you run. "
—Penny Chenery, in the movie *Secretariat*

WEEK 10: FEBRUARY 19, 2012
MONDAY—4 MILES EASY
TUESDAY— 5 X HILL, 2 DOWN
WEDNESDAY—4 MILES EASY
THURSDAY—9 MILES TEMPO
FRIDAY—REST
SATURDAY—5K RACE (OPTIONAL)
SUNDAY—20 MILES LONG EASY

One of the nice things about my entry into Boston is that I get regular email updates from the Boston Athletic Association, the race organizer. In this week's update was a picture of Desiree Davila. She stayed behind the pack biding her time. Desiree Davila chose to run her own race and ended up finishing second, just seconds behind the winner. I wondered what was going through her mind when she saw the pack of runners break away, what doubts.

Wise runners learn not to go out too fast in any race, especially a marathon, because they might not finish. They run at a pace and ability they can sustain for 26.2 miles.

It takes real courage to run your own race, whether it the Boston marathon, a local 5K, or making a decision in your everyday life. Sometimes it's tough to stay the course when you aren't sure it's the right decision.

Almost every time I run a marathon or even a half-marathon, I often ask myself "Why I am doing this?" Then I run the race and am always glad I did. I love to test myself and I can't do that if I don't run.

If you've finished a marathon, you know the exhilaration of running the best you can to conquer the distance. As a runner with CMT, I know I run a greater risk of being injured, but if I don't push myself, I would never know how far I can go. If I don't take a risk, I would never have set the goal of running Boston. Yet in 49 days, I will be lining up with thousands of other runners to do just that.

I'm doing quite a bit of questioning this week. Work is tough and has been exceptionally stressful. Sometimes "running my own race" at work separates me from my peers. I know the feeling of running alone. I know I've made the right decisions and done the right things. Sometimes running your own race means taking a risk even when there is no pay-off on the horizon. I'm not sure of the outcome, but am willing to live with the results.

The training got tough, too. On Thursday, I fell off the no-headset wagon and used the radio for my 9-mile tempo run. I was tired and since I had given up soda for Lent, I couldn't rely on the caffeine and sugar boost. So I cheated a bit by listening to talk radio and got the workout done. I didn't have a choice of moving the run to a later day because we were expecting rain and snow the next day.

I planned a 20-mile run for this weekend and was determined to run it outside. Saturday's temps were in the 20s. I was tired, so I pushed the run off until Sunday when the high was supposed to be 40F. Well, it was 28F when I got started and winds were predicted to hit 30 mph with gusts up to 45mph. I got out as early as possible to get at least part of my almost 4-hour run done before the winds were at their worst.

The run did not start out well when the bathrooms at the lake and in a nearby park were all locked. I had to make a pit stop at home, which messed up all my route plans. I only finished about 90 minutes of my run, and was feeling some pain in my right knee. It felt just like the pain I had when I got a stress fracture. My hamstrings were hurting and I was deter-mined to get through the workout without music.

Did I mention the wind? 40F sounds warm until you have 40-mph wind gusts. So I told myself to just run around the block and see how it goes. I wanted to be close to home in case I needed to stop.

I read a trick in a running magazine that I tried out as I ran the block. The article said when things get tough, to take your mind off the challenge, repeat a phrase like "left, right, left, right." So I started counting every step, 1,2,3,4,....until I got to 100. Then I started again. I counted off the 100-batches on my fingers until got to 1000. Then I repeated that five times and switched to another block. There were even a few hills.

My concentration was so powerful that I did not feel any pain. The counting pushed every other thought out of my head.

I watched the minutes tick off my running watch until I reached 3 hours and 50 minutes, my goal time for the workout.

Counting also helped me maintain a faster pace later in my workout. Every time I run one of these long workouts, I find it hard to believe on race day, I will have to run another hour. I wonder if I will ever make it.

The decision I made today will pay dividends when I run Boston. On a really tough day I was able to get through the workout. These are the small pieces that have to be in place. If it gets tough, I'll count or do whatever it takes...that's what it takes to run my race.

My legs feel good after today's workout. I'm still fighting a few trouble spots and I hope new running shoes this week will help. So whatever tough choices or decisions you have to make, do it. You won't know how far you can go unless you do.

Chapter 43
Breaking Barriers

Act as if what you do makes a difference. It does.
—William James, American philosopher and psychologist

Forty-five years ago, Katherine Switzer did something no other woman had ever done before. She registered and ran the Boston Marathon in 1967. Bobbi Gibbs had run the race a few years earlier, but was not registered and was not an official runner. Officials tried to pull Katherine off the course because women were not allowed. It was thought at one time running anything more than 10K was dangerous for women. Women were thought to be too fragile to run a marathon. She finished in 4 hours and 20 minutes.

Women lobbied the Amateur Athletic Union and in 1972, women were allowed to enter the Boston Marathon, but they had to meet the same time standard as men. Now the Boston Marathon field is made up almost half women.

I was in 8th grade the first year women were allowed in. At my school, there was no girls' cross-country team, only boys. The first girl joined the team in 1976—the year I graduated—and her presence was considered an oddity.

Katherine Switzer's run inspired other women to take up the sport and sparked a fitness and running revolution. She gave other woman the chance to put one foot in front of the other and run a race of their own. Every woman toeing the line in Boston or any marathon owes her an enormous debt.

Breaking a barrier—like entering a race—may seem like a small thing. I think it helped to pave changes for women in society and in the workplace. Acts like this gave women the courage to overcome numerous other personal and professional challenges as well.

I've been busy breaking barriers of my own. I graduated from college with a chemical engineering degree at the time when only about two percent of engineers were women. That number is still less than ten percent. So like Katherine, I'm living and thriving in a man's world.

Often, I am the only woman at the table during meetings. I know the feeling of someone trying to pull me off the course. Sometimes it's tough trying to break into the old boys club. I know all about doing things no one expects and exceeding expectations.

I'm breaking barriers for CMT as well. When I went to the Sports Medicine Clinic at a local hospital, the head of Physical Therapy told my therapist she did not know of any treatments for runners with CMT, because people with CMT can't run.

Well, obviously, some of us can and do run. People on Team CMT who can't run, swim or ride their bikes in events. I hope we are breaking our own barriers by showing those in the CMT community to be as active as their conditions allow.

While I may not be the first person with CMT to run Boston, I may be the first one to do it so publicly. I'm also running for people who have other invisible disabilities, like Lupus and Crohn's.

I hope that by giving a face to CMT, we can spark a revolution of our own. No one should carry a disease others have never heard of. No one should be told he or she shouldn't or can't be active. Many of us live with conditions no one can see that present daily challenges. We each choose how to react to our conditions.

Katherine didn't know the impact she would have when she ran her race—but she certainly made a big one for women's sports. She paved the way for athletes like Joan Benoit, who won the first women's Olympic Marathon in 1980.

Here's to Katherine and here's to breaking barriers.

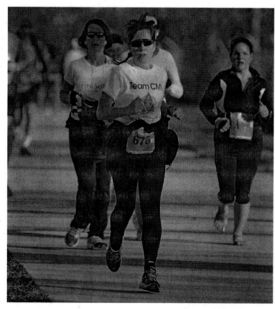

Breaking barriers—My debut race for HNF, Denton half-marathon, Dec. 31, 2011.

Chapter 44

Week 11: Training for Boston My New Best Friends

There is no satisfaction without a struggle first.
—Marty Liquori , athlete, broke the 4-minute mile in high school

WEEK 11: FEBRUARY26, 2012
MONDAY—5 MILES EASY
TUESDAY—6 X 800, 400 JOG
WEDNESDAY— 5 MILES EASY
THURSDAY—9 MILES TEMPO
FRIDAY—REST
SATURDAY—8 MILES PACE
SUNDAY—20 MILES LONG EASY

This was definitely a week of struggle. After my Sunday long run of 20+ miles, I couldn't walk without pain on Monday. My right Achilles tendon was so tight it hurt and no amount of stretching fixed it. I also had pain in both knees. There is a muscle right next to the knee cap, just to the inside of the legs, that on my right leg often gives me problems. Well, now both legs had muscle pain.

The good news it isn't a stress fracture; I was familiar with that type of pain since I had gotten a stress fracture while training for my first marathon. Since the pain was on both sides and got better with Biofreeze® , I knew it was in the muscles.

So this week Biofreeze® and Ibuprofen became my new best friends. Both are good for pain and inflammation from overuse. I also made two visits to my awesome chiropractor, Dr. Mark Drewicz. Treatment included ultrasound, muscle stimulation, and adjustments, all done twice. Dr. Mark treats many of the local long-distance runners and tri-athletes. I was referred to him by a runner friend. Dr. Mark has also been very supportive of Team CMT. He has given out dozens of promotional pens with the Team CMT website address and lets me put out fundraising fliers at his office.

I had to adjust my workouts a bit due to the injuries as well. I reduced my speed workout by 10 minutes and changed my 9-mile tempo run to a 9-mile easy run.

The right knee was still a little sore after a night of skiing on Saturday. I went to bed with an ice pack, an application of Biofreeze®, and a couple of Ibuprofen.

Sunday was 28F and snowing. We got 4 inches of wet snow on Friday night. I did not want to take a chance on slipping on the ice or of my injury getting worse. I decided to do a treadmill workout so I could stop if the knee got too bad.

It took a few ibuprofen and a couple of applications of Biofreeze® To get through the workout. I even did hill intervals to simulate the Boston course. 1.5 hours flat, 1.5 hours of increasing incline to simulate the 10 miles of rolling hills, and 6 minutes of high incline to simulate Heartbreak Hill. The workout was finished in 4 hours and 20 minutes. I feel good with no pain. I guess tomorrow will be the real test.

When you're fighting an injury, there is a fine line between trying to work through the injury and over-training. I've learned how to adapt my workouts to keep going when these injuries pop up. This week, I had to move my rest day from Friday to Wednesday to help me heal. I don't think I have ever gotten through an entire 18-week training program without a couple of injuries. It's still a mental hurdle when an injury threatens to put you out of the race. Looks like this time I may have beaten it.

This week also saw the debut of the Team CMT page on the HNF site. Allison and her team did a really great job. Be sure to check it out. You can also set up your own profile and fundraising page. www.hnf-cure.org

It turns out this week was an easy one. That's a relative term. An easy week at this point is a 6-mile tempo run, a 12-mile-long run and 5 miles on the other days. I get a rest day as well. I'll also be meeting my new coach this week. He will be helping me to get ready for Nationals in Austin at the end of May.

All in all, I feel satisfied and tired—a good and satisfied tired. I'm one week closer to Boston and feeling strong. I know I'll be ready.

Chapter 45
It Was All About a Boy

Sometimes our lack of confidence keeps us from trying
things we could easily master if we could summon
up the courage to get started.
—Tony Stoltzfus, Christian leadership coach

During our interview, local Milwaukee reporter Tom Held asked why I started running. I told him I started running to become a better skier. What he didn't ask was why I started skiing—it was all about a boy.

A college boy, actually. I was an 18-year-old freshman, just pledged to the Alpha Omicron Pi sorority at the University of Wisconsin in Milwaukee. One of my sorority sisters was dating a member of the engineering fraternity, Triangle. I was meeting her up in the Triangle office and as I was walking in, he was walking out. It was love at first sight...well, for me, anyway.

We'll call him Mr. Engineer. I later found out that Mr. Engineer was the object of most of my sorority sisters' crushes. Never mind, we had lots in common because we both worked as chemical lab technicians for local companies. He was a Chemical Engineering student and I was majoring in Chemistry, since I had started my college life as a pre-med major.

After a couple of semesters, I switched to engineering and was asked to join the engineering fraternity. Mr. Engineer was in charge of my training, so I got to see him quite a bit. One day, I worked up the courage to ask him to my sorority fall formal. He said no and it didn't even bother me. I was so excited that I actually had the courage to ask him. I had taken the risk and felt a lot of pride in myself. It was the feeling I still get every time I take a risk. Like the time I jumped off a cliff into the ocean in Kauai, Hawaii. The exhilaration was intoxicating.

I found out soon afterward that Mr. Engineer was a skier. Several of his frat brothers were heading to a local ski hill and invited my friend Ginny and me along. Since it was their first night skiing for the season, they dumped us on the bunny hill with no instruction. I spent the whole night getting up and falling down, but I was hooked.

I took a few lessons and improved my skiing skills enough to ski many nights and quite a few vacations skiing with Mr. Engineer, his frat brothers, and our mutual friends. He did everything well, including skiing. If athletic grace were a term in the dictionary, his picture would be next to it.

I have never been a natural athlete at anything. Friend Lynette was a little sister of the Triangle fraternity and a runner. When she invited me to go running, I knew it was the ticket to improve my skiing. It just so happened that Mr. Engineer was also a runner and Lynette and I would just happen to work out at the university track while Mr. Engineer and his buddy were running. I thought that if he just saw me, he would be smitten.

Not so much, since I looked about 12 years old when I was in college. He would have been a pedophile had he been attracted to me.

Well, Mr. Engineer never did fall in love with me. I eventually got over my crush and we became really good friends. He now lives in Boston, has been married for 20 years, and has two beautiful children. Hoping to connect with him in a few weeks.

* * * * *

You never know what influence your life may have on someone just by doing the things you do or what will happen if you are brave enough to take a risk.

My mom had been afraid to take risks. When she wanted to go to college, her dad said no, she should get a job until she got married. She had wanted to be a lawyer, but did not want to take the risk to oppose her dad. My dad told me the exact same thing when it was my time to go to college. I took the risk and went to school anyway and I am glad I did.

So be brave and take that risk, whether it's asking someone out, jumping off a cliff, pointing your skis downhill, or applying to the Boston Marathon. Think big and be brave.

Chapter 46

Week 12: Training for Boston Almost Famous

The Emperor Hadrian once said while building the Roman Empire, "Brick by brick, my citizens, brick by brick."

WEEK 12: MARCH 4, 2012
MONDAY—5 MILES EASY
TUESDAY— 6 X HILL, 2 DOWN
WEDNESDAY— 5 MILES EASY
THURSDAY—6 MILES TEMPO
FRIDAY—REST
SATURDAY—10K RACE (SUGGESTED)
SUNDAY—20 TO25 K

Rome wasn't built in a day and training for a marathon is not an overnight process either. You get ready workout by workout. It takes 18 weeks to build the stamina and endurance to cover the 26 miles. This week, I got a break because it was an easy week. The mileage builds for two weeks and then is cut back in the third week to give the body a chance to rest. Sometimes training for a marathon seems never-ending. It is just week after week of exhausting workouts.

I really have to take it one week at a time and not look too far ahead. I have to trust the training plan and know I will get not only to the starting line, but the finish line as well.

My long run was only 20 K, or 12 miles. Seemed easy since it only took 2 hours and 12 minutes. That was half the time of my longest run. I'm still fighting a couple of injuries but hanging in there. I often adjust my workouts. This week's schedule called for a 10 K race. Well, there is not always a race available locally so I substitute a 10K tempo run.

It was a busy and eventful week for Team CMT. My interview with a local TV station aired throughout the day on March 8th. I had complete strangers come up to me in the gym and tell me they had seen it. People have been asking lots of questions. Someone even told me he was inspired by my words. Hope he is inspired to work out. I haven't watched the video. I don't like to see myself in pictures or hear the sound of my own voice. Besides I was there, so I kind of already know what is in the interview.

The power of the media to reach out is worth all the effort to gain media attention. In just a few interviews, I've reached thousands through TV, newspaper, and radio. In just a few moments with reporters I've been able to bring awareness of CMT to thousands in the Milwaukee and Boston area. I knew the story of someone with CMT running the Boston Marathon would gain attention and it has. That makes all the pain and fatigue that come with training all worth it.

This week also brought some tremendous news. A donor in Boston is going to match donations for the Marathon run up to $10,000. I had pledged to raise $10,000 for HNF and wasn't even close yet. So I laid it on God and asked about the $10,000. Well, Thursday was when we got the large donation. In the future I should think bigger and ask for more.

If I can raise $10,000 and it is matched, I will have doubled the money I've invested in starting Team CMT and publicizing our efforts. Not a bad return.

Bit by bit, "brick by brick," we grow this team, raise money for research, and get ready for Boston.

This week, I have a 10K race with Team CMT members, an interview with Boston radio station, and a 20-mile-long run.

* * * * *

Raising awareness is just as important as raising money. Everyone watching my interview will learn about CMT. People don't give money for research for a disease they have never heard of. They give because they know a friend, family member, or co-worker with CMT. So raising awareness means raising money. Research costs money so every dollar raised is needed.

Raising awareness is important for those with CMT. It is bad enough to have a disease, and even worse when you get a blank stare when you tell someone about it. It is like being a victim twice. Raising awareness helps us disclose our condition to others.

It gets exhausting trying to explain about CMT every time I tell someone I have it. Once in a while, I meet someone familiar with CMT and it is such a relief. I think that is why there is such a bond between people on Team CMT. There are others who have heard of CMT and understand it. No need for any explanation. I know some people with CMT who just say they have MS, because they get that nod of recognition and they don't have to give a big explanation.

I don't take that route. Every person I tell about my CMT is one more person I have educated, even if that means I will be treated differently. I would like to tell others in the CMT community take the same approach. Many do not talk about their CMT and some even seem ashamed of having CMT. None of us with this condition have anything to be ashamed of. We did not do anything to get CMT; we were born with it. It is part of who we are. It is part of what we experience every day.

I am starting to see a slight shift in the Facebook groups about disclosure. I remember one man saying he wears braces and wears shorts in the summer so they are visible. He carries brochures with him explaining CMT when he is asked about his braces. I applaud that kind of courage. I hope we see more of it and I hope my efforts and those of Team CMT help open the way.

Each act is one more brick—whether on the road to the Boston Marathon, raising awareness, or finding treatments and a cure.

Chapter 47
The Best Advice I Ever Got

Most people give up just when they're about to achieve success.
They quit on the one yard line. They give up at the last minute
of the game, one foot from a winning touchdown.
—Ross Perot, American businessman

I was once asked during a job interview to relate the best advice I was ever given. It's a great question and an easy one for me to answer.

It was during engineering graduate school. I graduated during a terrible recession. I couldn't have bought a job. I even traveled to the East Coast at my own expense to interview.

I was working in a local department store to make ends meet when I finally landed a research job at a large international company with headquarters in Milwaukee. My job was to conduct research on the materials used to make humidity sensors for building control systems.

One of the requirements of my employer was that I return to graduate school, since the knowledge I needed to do this work was only taught at the master's level. I was happy to do so since I loved going to school. So I enrolled in a graduate program to study electronic materials. I worked full time and was taking 6 credits, or two classes. If I took 6 credits, payment of my undergraduate student loans would be deferred.

I had accumulated a small amount of debt when I quit working the last year of college to finish my degree. Getting an engineering degree can be an intense experience. I was doing a senior research project and taking several senior-level design courses in my Chemical Engineering program. There was so much homework I did all nighters every other night. That kind of work load just did not work with a part-time job. The loans I took out were not huge by today's standards, but starting out, I did not have much money. My tuition was paid by my company and the more courses I took in a semester, the more quickly I would graduate.

Taking two classes meant lots of homework. I spent most of my weekends reading and finishing off assignments so I would be ready for class. Still the workload was much lighter than my last year of undergraduate school and it seemed like a good trade-off. I was missing some short-term fun in hopes of advancing may career. It was a choice that was easy to make.

As part of my graduate program, I took a class in thermodynamics and used math to prove basic thermodynamic laws. I spent endless hours working out the equations. It isn't fun writing page after page of equations when you just aren't getting to the answer. It's even less fun when you see your friends head out the door to have fun at the bars.

Part of the course requirements was meeting with the professor to go over the homework. My professor had an unpronounceable Middle-Eastern name, so we'll just call him Professor K.

One day, when going over my assignment, Professor K said to me, "Christine, you get so close to solving the problem and then you stop."

I have always remembered that feedback. If I had just worked a little harder and stuck with it a little longer, I would have solved the problem—or so he thought. That really gave me something to think about. Was I quitting too soon? Was I giving up? If I worked a little longer and a little harder, would I have been successful? What if I didn't stop until I solved the problem?

What did this mean on a larger scale? I remember reading about Thomas Edison. He tried thousands of different materials until he found the right material to serve as a filament for his light bulb. His desire and his determination never to quit until he found the solution made him successful.

My professor's words echoed in my head as I ran my first marathon. I wanted to quit many times during that race. My thighs burned and blisters caused my feet to bleed all the way through my shoes. But I was no quitter. I was not quitter then and I am no quitter now.

I finished that first marathon in four hours and have finished five marathons since then. I'll finish marathon number seven when I line up for the Boston Marathon in April. Those same words and determination will get me to the finish line one more time.

I know no matter how tough it gets in a race, not to quit too soon. I've carried that same attitude into my entire life—whether it's a race, a project at work, or finding a cure for the condition I share with so many others. I know not to quit anything too soon, before that problem is solved, the project finished, and the finish line crossed.

Chapter 48
Week 13: Training for Boston
A Good Week

Running a marathon gave me the inner strength that
changed my life....just finishing can have a profound
effect on your confidence and self-esteem.
—Henley Gibble, Exec. Dir. of Road Runners Club of America

WEEK 13: MARCH 11, 2012
MONDAY—5 MILES EASY
TUESDAY—7 X 800, 400
WEDNESDAY—5 MILES EASY
THURSDAY—6 MILES TEMPO
FRIDAY—REST
SATURDAY—5 MILES EASY
SUNDAY—20 MILES LONG EASY, LUCK OF THE IRISH 10K

This week was full of accomplishments for Team CMT members nationally and locally. Virginia Team CMT member Ruth finished her first marathon at the Shamrock Marathon in Virginia Beach this weekend.

I still remember how great it felt when I finished my first marathon. After crossing the finish line, I knew there was nothing in life I wouldn't be able to accomplish. I feel that way every time I cross the finish line. Every mile is hard won and makes the accomplishment that much sweeter.

Sometimes I think getting through all the training is just as tough or maybe even a little tougher than running the race itself. I have been using the same training program for years from a *Runner's World* magazine article. I've customized it a bit due to my CMT, cross-training every other day instead of running. I usually train by myself because I am slow and because I can control the quality of my workouts much better that way. Unless someone is training for a marathon, he or she may not be running long enough or doing the same kind of speed workouts I am doing. There will be runners in Milwaukee training for Boston doing similar workouts, but they will be much, much faster than I am. So I train alone, mostly because my running speed is not a good match for most runners training for an event like Boston

I am glad Ruth knows what it feels like to finish a marathon and be among the one percent of Americans who have run a marathon. Ruth now joins Team CMT members Katie (who did her 2nd marathon as a Team CMT member this weekend), Richard, Mary, Kristin, Robert, Cheryl, and myself. Congratulations also to Pat for finishing the half-marathon and to Katie for finishing the marathon on a day when she was sick. Katie is trying to qualify for Boston so she can run with Richard next year. Get 'em next time, Katie!

Here in Wisconsin, we had the 10K "Luck of the Irish" Run in Hartland. I was joined by team members Robert, Cheryl Kathy and Lincoln.

My plan was to run the race easy to test my marathon pace. The 10K race was actually just the first part of my 20-mile Sunday. The course was three loops with two big hills in each loop. Everyone looked pretty tired and complained about the course when they finished. I ran the loop again to get the hill work in and add a little mental toughness. I finished it in one hour. That was good enough to give me the chance of running a 4:41 in Boston.

Cheryl took 4th for her age group in the race and won her age group for the series. There were awards for each race and everyone who raced at least five of the six races in the series was eligible for overall series awards. I took it easy and placed 9th. Lincoln took 4th in his age group.

Racing is fun and makes all the hard workouts worthwhile. I went home, took a nap, and ran 11 more miles later in the day. The knee was still hurting, but so far, I am getting through the workouts.

This week is the last week of long runs. It will be the second week in a row of a 10-mile tempo run and a 20-mile run. After this week, it's a taper to the finish. Boston is getting close. Training for a marathon can be summed up in three things: Run Hard, Recover, Repeat. Mileage builds for a few weeks and then there is a rest week. This gives the body a chance to adapt to the hard training workload. At this point in the training program, all the hard work to get my body ready for race day is done. Now is the recovery, right up until race day. It is all necessary part to be ready when I line up at the starting line. Almost there.

Chapter 49

Week 14: Training for Boston I'm Not Normal

Our lives are fashioned by choice. First we make choices.
Then our choices make us.
—Andy Andrews, speaker and author of *The Travelers' Gift*

WEEK 14 : MARCH 18, 2012
MONDAY—5 MILES EASY
TUESDAY—7 X HILL, 3 DOWN
WEDNESDAY—5 MILES EASY
THURSDAY—10 MILES TEMPO
FRIDAY—REST
SATURDAY—4 MILES MARATHON PACE
SUNDAY—20 MILES LONG EASY

This was the second week I had to do a 10-mile tempo run and a 20-mile run back to back weeks. It was foggy, rainy, and 50F on Saturday and my legs were stiff. My chiropractor, Dr. Drewicz, had advised me to do my long run on Sunday to give my sore knee an extra day off. I wanted to do the run on Saturday since I have a half-marathon the follow ing Saturday. Dr. Mark won the argument.

On Sunday, it was 52F and sunny when I started my 20-mile run in Lake Park along Lake Michigan. I needed a change to keep things fresh and wanted one last chance to run hills. I ran the long hill off of Kenwood, St Mary's Hill, and the hill by Alterra coffee all at least five times. The loop I ran was five miles long, but stairs, hills, and trail running in Lake Park made up the three hours. I finished my run with 30 minutes through some of Milwaukee's East Side, even passing my old flat on Shepherd. I am still running without music or radio, so I have plenty of time to think.

I've concluded that I'm not normal. As I passed both Lake Park Bistro and Cafe Hollander, it seemed like the whole East Side was either having brunch or waiting to be seated on the terrace. I got a good whiff of breakfast food at both places. Everyone was out golfing, roller-blading, drinking coffee at Alterra, walking their dog, or generally having a good time. There I was, doing hill after hill and stairs, banging out another

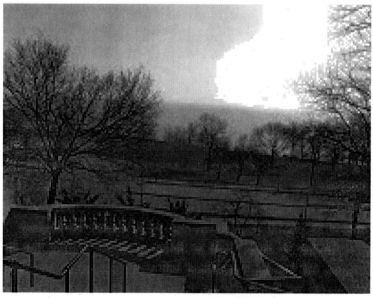

Lake Park stairs I ran to train for Boston

20-mile run. Sometimes it makes me a little sad and I wonder if I am missing out or if I've made the better choice.

It's still it my choice and it was a great day for a run. It feels good to have my last really long run done.

This run also made me think of some of the things I give up when I'm training for a marathon. It takes so much time to train, there is not much time left for anything else. My 20-mile runs take over four hours. My legs are so sore afterward that I don't feel up to anything except a nap.

I only get to the movies about once or twice a year or even watch movies at home or join friends for a Sunday brunch. It's all by choice and it will all be worth it when I line up on race day.

My cousin's daughter was just in her high school musical. I really wanted to go, but after a long run, my legs were just too sore and I was too tired. If I judge my success by what I have to give up to be ready for a marathon, then I am wildly successful.

I never do Happy Hour, between 4 and 6-ish on week-days. Fitting in dinner with friends is a challenge. I have to carefully plan to see them and still get in my workout for the day. The average person is okay if he or she works out only a few times a week. It takes working out 6 to 7 days a week for me to be ready for an event like Boston. I am taking the spot of someone else who wants to be there as much as I do. I owe that anonymous person a hard and steady effort. I train out of respect for myself as an athlete and out of respect for the race.

In just 21 days, I will be lining up on the starting line in Boston. All that fun I sacrificed will really pay off on race day. So maybe my Sunday is not "normal" for the average person, but it's par for the course of any serious athlete. It's a choice I gladly make to be ready for the biggest race I've ever run.

It was a good week. I met with Tom Held of the *Milwaukee Journal-Sentinel* for an interview. I talked so much, I'm surprised he came back for the photo shoot on Thursday. Tom is a runner, skier, and cyclist, so it was great to meet him. He asked a number of questions that showed he'd read my blog, which I really appreciated. It is a great honor to be interviewed by Tom. He has done profiles on a number of local runners, including two pieces on my elite runner ex-boyfriend. I know I've arrived when I've been interviewed by Tom Held. I really appreciated his time.

The weeks get easier now. I'm on my taper on training. Mileage is gradually decreased up to the race. This means all the hard work is done. Now I just have to let me body rest and repair. I love the taper, which includes two days off in the days just before the race. My longest run this week will be the Trailbreaker Half-marathon next Saturday in Waukesha, but I will run it if the knee feels good. The legs really hurt today during the run and I always wonder how I will do 26 when 20 miles hurt so much. Of course, on race day, I will take liberal doses of Ibuprofen. That and a little race day magic will get me to the finish.

Chapter 50
It Takes a Team

Win or lose, you will never regret working hard, making sacrifices, being disciplined or focusing too much. Success is measure by what we have done to prepare for competition.
—Jon Smith, British author

I t takes a team to get to the marathon starting line healthy and ready to race. I read that twenty percent of those registered for the New York Marathon got injured and didn't make it to the starting line. Hard work and dedication only get you so far.

Keeping an athlete with CMT healthy is quite a challenge and I have a great team of medical professionals helping me get ready to compete. Our condition makes injury a common part of our experience. A good team to deal with injuries and maybe even prevent them is essential to my success as a runner and triathlete.

My team includes a great chiropractor, physical therapist, sports medicine physician, as well as researchers who are looking for a cure for CMT, and a number of others.

To compete at the national level, I needed advice and accountability. I am consistent in my training, but reporting on my progress helps me to stay that way. I also like having a second opinion on my training plans.

I tried using a local coach. I explained my goals for Boston and triathlon competition at the national level. In our initial meeting, I explained I could not run every day due to my CMT. In the first week, he gave me workouts with consecutive days of running. I reminded him I could not do that without getting injured. When he did it a third time within that same month, he became an ex-coach.

I then approached Florida USAT Level 1 Triathlon Coach Joy Von Werder. She is an Ironman finisher—and she has CMT. I don't have to explain anything to her. As an athlete, she knows what I go through. I email her every day. Joy has been with me through injuries and all the up and downs of being a CMT-affected athlete. She is my coach, advocate, and fellow Team CMT member.

I so appreciate the advice and expertise of all these professionals. I hope they feel I am worthy of their time and attention.

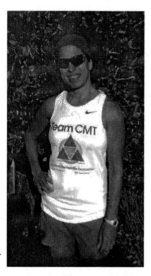

My coach Joy Von Werder

Chapter 51
Week 15: Training for Boston
Tapering is Tough

God moves mountains to create the opportunity of
His choosing. It is up to you to be ready to move yourself.
—Andy Andrews, motivational speaker and coach

WEEK 15: MARCH 25, 2012
MONDAY—5 MILES EASY
TUESDAY—8 X 800, 400
WEDNESDAY—5 MILES EASY
THURSDAY—8 MILES TEMPO
FRIDAY—REST
SATURDAY—5 MILES MARATHON PACE
SUNDAY—20 MILES LONG EASY

It's starting to get real now, because my participant packet arrived on Friday afternoon. Just two weeks from Monday, I will be lining up with over 27,000 other runners. I wish it was here already, because the waiting is tough. Too much time to think about the race.

I'm now in the taper phase of my training. After weeks of intense speed work and long runs, the workouts are drastically cut back. This gives the body time to rest and repair to be ready for the rigors of racing 26.2 miles.

While the reduction in mileage is nice, it can be a mental adjustment when you are used to the tough workouts. Now the mental second-guessing starts. Did I run enough and am I ready for the hills in Boston? Did I do the right things to be ready for the initial stretch of ten miles downhill? How will I feel on race day? Can I fight the pain and fatigue to finish? Will people be disappointed in me?

I had lots of time to think about the race on Friday night. Friday was one of those nights where I struggled all night to fall asleep. Fight is a good word for it. After two hours of tossing and turning, I got up and took two Tylenol PM, then two over-the-counter sleep tablets an hour later. I repeated this with more sleep aid and Tylenol at various times. At 3:45 a.m., I gave in and took a prescription sleeping pill. Why had I waited so long? I try to save the prescription meds for when I am really desperate, so I don't build up a tolerance for them. It was a tough night because my whole body was jumpy and felt like it was on fire, so I am pretty sure this is CMT-related.

After four hours of sleep, I turned off the alarm that was supposed to wake me up for the half-marathon race I had scheduled in Waukesha. I could have run. I know I can run on little sleep, I just didn't think it was a good idea so close to Boston.

I bounced back Sunday and got my 12-mile run in on the treadmill since it was 42F and rainy. It felt so good I didn't want to stop. It is a big temptation during the taper to do just a bit more to get ready. The rest before is just as important as all the tough workouts.

Another bright spot this week was Tom Held's article in the *Milwaukee Journal-Sentinel.* Tom actually got a decent picture of me, which is quite a feat.

I know that despite my doubts, I have prepared harder for this race than I have for any of my previous six marathons. I know I've done my best. We'll just have to wait until race day to see if it was enough.

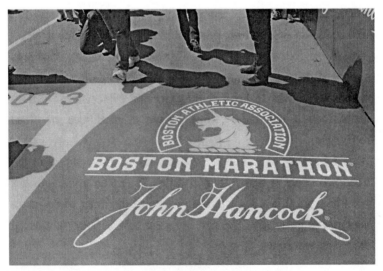

The Boston finish line—the goal for which I was training so hard.

Chapter 52
Race Drama

Success without adversity is not only empty...it is not possible.
—General H. Norman Schwarzkopf

J ust a bit of drama for me as I line up for the Boston Marathon on race day. I've had a finish line fantasy for quite some time. I always dreamt my significant other would meet me as I completed those final tough miles or at least be at the finish line.

There won't be any hero in Boston. No significant other in my life at the moment. I've only had spectators at one marathon. My brother and his girlfriend were at the Madison finish line and friend Cheryl cheered me on from our hotel steps in Madison.

No finish line hero in Boston—just an ex-boyfriend running in the elite wave. I thought he'd be my finish line hero. While we dated, I heard all his stories about training for and running Boston. He has run Boston more than twenty times and is well known in local running circles. He has won several of the local marathons numerous times, and helped me get ready for my first marathon when I ran my best time. His success fueled my interest.

We had been friends for more than ten years before we started dating. He also helped me get through being unemployed and was always a source of advice on running and injuries. He was always able to give me a referral for a doctor, massage therapist, or chiropractor. We would talk for hours. He knew I was interested in him and I was ready when he suggested we start dating.

I called him my "light-bulb boyfriend," off, then on, then off— always at his whim. Each "on" time, I took him back because when you hit the 40-year mark, it's pretty tough to find a decent guy, and, well, I was in love. He would look all sorry and look at me with his big blue eyes and I would melt. I saw a little boy who only wanted to be loved. I would want someone to take me back if the tables were turned.

I knew I wasn't the love of his life, but thought if I just worked hard enough, was understanding enough, and be a good enough girlfriend, I would win him over. I thought if I hung in there long enough, things would work out. I had waited so long to date him, I didn't want to give up too soon. He was everything I wanted. Even as the years wore on, I was as excited to be with him as I had been at the beginning of our time together.

We had a fight one day and did not talk for months. When we did talk, he told me he was seeing someone else and dropped out of my life for two years.

Then he dropped back in. We were in "just friends" status. He told me he had broken up and the ex-girlfriend was kind of "psycho." He also said he had been seeing a single mom and she just did not have the time to spend with him. It all seemed very believable.

I was not seeing anyone, and although I had not been waiting around for him to come back, we were back "on."

We did not see each other as much as I would have liked. But two demanding careers, sick parents, and training schedules all seemed like logical explanations. We saw each other pretty often all things considered. We dated or two years until my birthday, when he suggested lunch. I lost it. I felt like I was being put in the "friend" category. I told him I was tired of being an afterthought in his life while he looked for someone else. He rang my phone off the hook trying to get me back. He called every week. He was trying to work his way back into my life, even suggesting I go to Prague with him to visit his brother, who was there on a long-term work assignment.

A few days later, I got an email that changed my life. It was from the supposedly ex-girlfriend. It turned out he had never broken up with her and had been seeing both of us, and was actually living with her, making me the other woman. I had even spent time in his house. Guess I should have looked in the closets and cabinets. Once, when my sister came home for Dad's 75th birthday, we all met at the boyfriend's house before going out to dinner. My sister said he looked like he was acting kind of guilty. I put it down to being a bit awkward meeting some of my family.

I think when the girlfriend emailed me, it was not just a friendly gesture. She was trying to tell me to stay away from her man. Too bad I didn't know she was still in the picture. I never would have spent any time with him had I known. I suspect he knew, too, or he would not have lied about his status for two years. I think he knew I would not want to be part of hurting someone else.

From piecing things together, I figured out this was not the first time he had "double booked" himself. He had done it to us both before. He was dating me when he met her. I believe it was over two years that time. Honestly, I don't know how he made the time for both of us, because I was seeing him fairly often. It is a wonder he never got caught.

I haven't talked with him since that fall afternoon. I was angry and let him know I did not want him to ever come around again asking to get back together. I could not be sure I would not be weak again, so I wanted to be certain it was the last thought on his mind.

I do see him occasionally at runs, but try to avoid events I think he will run and have switched mostly to triathlons, which makes it easier.

His name has come up a lot lately. My chiropractor is friends with him and mentions him most visits, and Tom Held, brought up his name during our interview. My hair stylist asked if that runner dude was still with "that woman." I did a little poking around on the Internet, and, yes, he is engaged to the woman who emailed me.

That news hit me a bit hard. It doesn't seem fair that he gets to be happy. He lied to me, took advantage of my feelings for him, and used me to hurt someone else. She was so anxious to warn me away from her man that she didn't care that she hurt me. She does not seem to mind he had double-dipped before. She invaded my privacy emailing me and even calling my house.

That fall afternoon, I lost I thought had been my best friend. I lost all my hopes and dreams for things working out with him, and lost any good memories I had of my time with him because now I think I was always just someone on the side. Maybe they both deserve each other, because if you're in a relationship and reading his work and personal emails, you don't trust him. If you don't trust him, you have no business making a lifelong commitment. He won't change because he put a ring on your finger. If he cheated during the bloom of love, an engagement or even a marriage won't change that. You can't build a happy life on the ashes of someone else's. And yes, in this case, he will cheat again. He never even said he was sorry to me for what he did. Maybe he isn't sorry. In fact, at a run last year, he flirted up a storm with a little red-haired woman. So I don't think he is a changed man or has learned anything from the experience.

I have my own family experience to draw from. My dad repeatedly cheated on my mom. The one who was the last straw was a 19-year-old he met in a bar. She was just a few years older than my sister; Dad was in his 50s. It was not the first time my dad cheated, but it was the last time my mom tolerated it. She had tried to preserve her marriage for the sake of her kids. So while she was home taking care of the kids, he was giving out his number to barflies young enough to be his daughter. I know all about the fling through the magic of Facebook.

The barfly posted all the details. Some people have no shame. She knew he was married. I guess that does not matter to some people. This same woman followed my dad when he retired to northern Wisconsin. She and her daughter were able to persuade my dad to give them loans for all of the money he had. When he went into a nursing home, nothing was left for his care. So I guess what goes around, comes around. My dad is paying the price for his actions, but it still affects us because the rest of the family is left to pick up the pieces. I hope people don't think that when they cheat, they aren't hurting anyone. The hurt is deep and profound. It changes lives and relationships.

My runner friend knew of this family history and how it affected me. He knew it was something I would not tolerate. We talked about it several times. I hope my ex at some point in his life feels even a fraction of the pain he has caused me and the other women in his life. That would be justice to me. It is what I hold on to.

After a good night's sleep and a run, I was OK. Everything always feels better after a run.

Hopefully this experience gets me one step closer to that finish line hero I'm still looking for. Maybe next time, I will be wiser. With CMT and being over 50, it's a lot to hope for, but I'm a optimistic romantic.

Chapter 53

Week 16: Training for Boston
A Near Miss

It's not whether you get knocked down; it's whether you get up.

—Vince Lombardi

WEEK 16: APRIL 1, 2012
MONDAY—5 MILES EASY
TUESDAY—8 X HILL, 3 DOWN
WEDNESDAY—5 MILES EASY
THURSDAY—6 MILES TEMPO
FRIDAY—REST
SATURDAY—4 MILES MARATHON PACE
SUNDAY—12 MILES LONG EASY

I told my friend and HNF president, Allison Moore, early this week that I was healthy and injury free. I would be at the starting line unless I had a fall or an accident. I think it was bad luck to even say such a thing.

I did have a fall and came close to being hit by a car. I was bike shopping on the East Side of Milwaukee. Parking is tight there so I had to park across from the bike shop. It wasn't open and I had to cross the traffic-filled street a second time to get back to my car. I guessed I could dash across before the next car arrived. I should have known better.

Halfway across, I suddenly found myself on my hands and knees with a car coming straight at me. I hadn't accounted for falling time in my calculations. I'm not sure why the driver never got close enough to hit me. He or she must have slowed enough to let me get up and finish my trip across the street. It's scary to fall without warning. It is part of my CMT and happens when I least expect it.

I have a bump on each knee and nice red spots. The palms of my hands are pretty tender as well. Later that afternoon, my right knee got pretty stiff and I had trouble walking. A little ice and it was as good as new.

I don't seem any worse for the wear. I always joke that I fall a lot, but God blessed me with rubber bones. So despite the near miss, I'm still on track for Boston. It's only eight days away.

Training was pretty quiet this week. I did my last long run of eight miles today. It seemed easy. It was 54F and windy. A perfect day for a run. I often do errands on my long runs. Doing so gets me out the door. Today it was a trip to the post office to mail bills and a trip to the ATM to deposit a couple of checks. Nice to combine the two. The time went by quickly. No music on this run. In fact, except for one workout, the music ban has held up. I still plan on running Boston iPod-free.

The workouts this coming week are pretty easy, nothing longer than a 4-mile run. Friday and Saturday are off days, and Sunday is a 3-mile run. I leave for Boston on Friday.

Let's hope for a safer and fall-free week this week. No more near misses, even though I am good at getting up when I fall. I guess one of the keys in life is getting back up when you fall, whether it's a setback at work, a failed romance, or literally hitting the street with a car bearing down on you.

I'm ready for Boston physically and emotionally. Can't wait to get to Boston and meet our Team CMT members there. I'm excited and as the race gets closer, I'll be a little nervous. I'm really looking forward to the fundraiser and running the race.

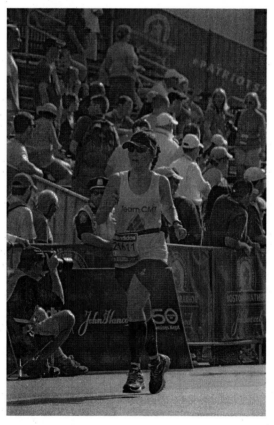

What I was working for ...

Chapter 54
Self-Inflicted Injury

The difference between perseverance and obstinacy
is that one comes from a strong will
and the other comes from a strong won't.
—Henry Ward Beecher, American social reformer

I t takes a strong will to prepare for a marathon. Whether the goal is to run well or finish, you have to be consistent in your training. You have to run when you're tired, had a bad day at work, or when fighting injuries.

While training for Boston, I fought a number of injures, first to my Achilles tendons in both legs and then my knees. The knee injury was on the muscle on the medial part of the knee and it was on both knees. That was really unusual, because my injuries always happen on my right leg. It's where I got the stress fracture training for my first marathon. The right Achilles tendons is always tight and hurts.

So it was surprising when both knees had a problem. I was still able to keep training, but it was puzzling that they were not only not getting better, but a bit worse. One day, my chiropractor was asking me all kinds of questions about my shoes and my orthotics. I had changed shoes, but was using the same model. I had only been running on them for a month.

Many runners wear custom-made inserts in their shoes called orthotics. The inserts are custom designed for each runner's foot taken from plaster casts. The orthotics put the runner's foot into a neutral position. Most runners' feet either roll inward or outward when they run, causing injuries. The orthotics allow the foot to stay level as the athlete runs, preventing injuries. I could not run without them because of my CMT and in addition, I have really high arches. The orthotics support my feet and make up for some of the issues my feet have due to my CMT.

I know my orthotics were good. They were designed by Dr. Barczak, a former All-American runner. All Dr. Mark's questions made me pull out my running shoes when I got home.

I pulled out the inserts to look at them and discovered I had them in the wrong shoes—the right orthotic was in the left shoe, and vice versa.

You would think I would be able to feel that, but I couldn't. There is s test the neurologist does at my yearly appointment. He takes a needle and pricks the skin, starting at the foot and going to the knee. I know a pin is pricking me but I can barely feel it. So no, I can't tell when my inserts are in the wrong shoes.

The knee injury was self-inflicted. Once I got my running shoes set up correctly, the knee problem went away.

This is not the first time I have done something like this. Twice this year while on ski patrol, I put my boots on the wrong feet. The sensation a normal person has to tell them that is wrong just doesn't work for me anymore. That was embarrassing because the second time it happened, one of my fellow patroller's saw it. We had a good laugh about.

I laughed about it too because it is funny, but it is also serious as well. It could have cost me a chance to run at Boston if I had not corrected the problem with the orthotics . It is also a reminder that my disease is marching on. There is no running away from that, no matter how much I train.

Right now, the strong will is still winning and the strong won't is helping to find a solution to every problem CMT presents. It won't stop me from running Boston at least not this time.

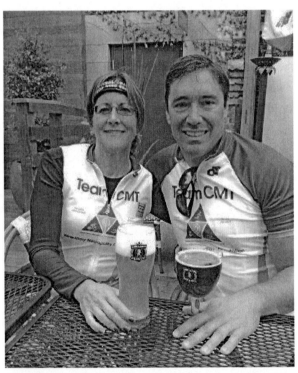

Original Team CMT members, Cheryl Monnat and Robert Kearney

Chapter 55

Week 17: Training for Boston Rested and Ready

A winner's strongest muscle is her heart.
—Cassie Campbell, Canadian ice hockey player

WEEK 17: APRIL 8, 2012
MONDAY— 5 MILES EASY
TUESDAY—4 X 800, 400
WEDNESDAY—3 MILES EASY
THURSDAY—4 MILES TEMPO
FRIDAY— REST — OFF TO BOSTON!
SATURDAY—REST
SUNDAY—2 MILES EASY

I arrived safely in Boston and was as ready as I could be for race day on Monday. Team member Trenni will also be wearing a Team CMT singlet. Trenni was the TV reporter who did a story about my CMT and my Boston run. It was really nice of her to agree to be on the team.

All the training is done. Now it's just three days until race day and I am nervous and excited. Usually I am really nervous about running a marathon. Anything can happen on race day and with CMT I never know what part is going to hurt or if I will have enough energy to finish the race. I always wonder if the training I did was enough or if it was the right kind of training.

I am excited because I am realizing a long-held dream. I waited so long and worked so hard to get here. It is so great to be having two of us raising awareness of CMT on such a big stage.

It takes a big heart to run for a cause just because you were asked. So thanks, Trenni!

The weekend is also exciting because I will be connected with old friends and meeting new ones.

I will be visiting with an old college friend, touring his company, and having dinner with his family. He was the inspiration for my running career. Without his influence, I might never have become a runner.

College friend Cheryl Monnat and her boyfriend Robert Kearney will be joining me to be my entourage for the weekend.

A pre-event party organized by Boston Team CMT member Duane Denny is set up for Sunday night. Several Team CMT members I have never met will be coming and I can't wait to meet them. HNF president Allison Moore will be there, too. I'm so happy she will be on the course as well sharing in this event. I appreciate the support she has given me and the team throughout the process. The party is also a great opportunity to meet donor Gerald Lynch, who is matching contributions to the run. I will also be meeting his 10-year-old daughter, who has CMT.

With his donation, I was able to raise $10,000 to go toward CMT research and awareness raising activities.

It is going to be a packed and emotional weekend. I hope I can keep it all together as I cross the finish line. I get choked up just thinking about it. Over and over in my mind, I see myself finishing strong and running well all day. There is even a chance I could place within my division. Last year, my time would have been good enough for third. The top two runners are back this year. I wonder what it would be like to step up and accept my 3rd place award. I hope I make everyone proud.

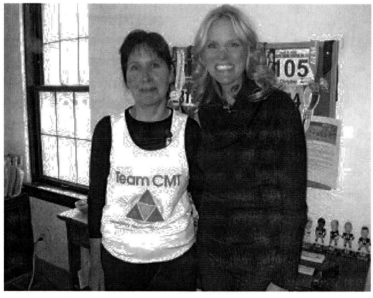

Trenni Kusnierek and me the day of my TV interview.

Chapter 56
Least Likely to Succeed

It's not who you are that's holding you back,
it's who you think you are.
—Denis Waitley, motivational speaker and author

I t was not all business when I was in Boston. I started the trip with a visit with my college friend, Viktor. We talked about my Boston Marathon run and the fact I would be competing at the National Triathlon Sprint Championship in Austin, Texas six weeks after Boston. He laughed and said I was the last person he would have expected going to a national competition. I chuckled and agreed. So while I was training for Boston, I was also aiming for Austin.

I was still trying to wrap my mind around the fact that if I place 1st in my in Austin, would gain a spot on the US team and have a chance to compete at the World Championship in New Zealand. At the Paratriathlon National Championships, athletes are placed in categories reflecting their disability. Those of us with neuromuscular conditions are classified as TRI 3. There are seven triathlon categories. I've come a long way from the girl who sat the bench for two years of grade-school volley ball and endured endless taunting about my slow running.

I've overcome lots of limitations by working hard. I had to do something even harder to get ready for Boston. I had to stop working out to let an ankle injury heal. I realize how much sports have become a part of my life and who I am. I had to put aside training and working out for four difficult days so I could get to Austin injury free.

I ran for the first time in weeks and it felt wonderful. I had put off doing triathlons for years because I was afraid of doing the open water swim. I panicked the first two races and had to do the backstroke to through the race, but I made it.

There are fears and doubts for this race, too. This is only my 5th triathlon and I still feel like a beginner. I have very little experience doing open water swims, and I'm still figuring out bike racing and transitions. Just hope I don't make any big mistakes and I get through the race.

I'll have tough competition. The current champion lives in Alabama and has probably been riding for months. I have had a few weeks to get used to my new clipless pedals. I will be competing against athletes who are younger and more experienced.

While training and racing, I used to wonder why I was not a better runner. I am so consistent in my workouts and work so hard. I've often thought I good be a really good athlete if I just had some talent. I often wondered why God made me so competitive, with so much desire to succeed, and then leave out the talent. Well, it turns out, He didn't. My friend Joyce, who also has CMT, always made me laugh when she said I was fast. Joyce is right—for someone with CMT, I am incredibly fast. My talent may be masked by CMT, but it is still there and apparent when I am measured against others with similar challenges. I never thought I would consider myself an elite athlete. I've learned to change that image of myself. I will be competing at the national level against the best athletes in the country. I am proud and thankful to be in such company.

Life is funny. You never know what unexpected opportunities will present themselves. The chance to compete in a national championship is one I never expected. I am going to make the most of it. I am so excited to be there and am going to have as much fun as possible and not worry about anything else. I'll remind myself how far I've come and what I've had to give up to get there. And I will try not to focus on how much I have yet to learn. If there is one thing I've learned: the biggest limitations people face are the ones they put on themselves.

Chapter 57
Week 18: Training for Boston
I'm Committed

Until one is committed
There is hesitancy, the chance to draw back
Always ineffectiveness.
Concerning all acts of initiative (and creation)
There is one elementary truth
The ignorance of which kills countless ideas
and splendid plans;
That the moment that one definitely commits oneself
Then Providence moves, too.
All sorts of things occur to help on
That would never have otherwise occurred.
A whole steam of events issues from the decision
Raising in one's favor all manner
Of unforeseen incidents and meetings
And material substance
Which no one could have dreamt
Would have come your way.
Whatever you can do or dream you can, begin it.
Boldness has genius, power and magic in it.
—Wolfgang Goethe

WEEK 18: APRIL 15, 2012
NO TRAINING THIS WEEK
MONDAY BOSTON MARATHON!!!!!!

When I was diagnosed with CMT in 2010, I set the goal of running the Boston Marathon to raise awareness and money for CMT research. Never mind that I'd given up competitive running, that I hadn't run a marathon in over ten years, and my CMT had left me far short of the qualifying time. Oh, and I am a slow, middle-aged woman with a neurological disease that makes running a challenge.

I wrote the date April 16, 2012 on a piece of paper and pinned it to my bulletin board at work. I told everyone I was going to Boston. I was committed. I didn't want to just run Boston; I wanted to represent those with CMT by wearing a Team CMT uniform. And I was going to tell the world about it, if it would listen.

Some truly amazing things have happened since I wrote down that goal.

When I couldn't get a CMT-based charity certified, I poked around the Boston Marathon website and stumbled onto the Mobility Impaired program. It's for athletes with conditions that keep them from making the time standard. While the B.A.A. had never heard of CMT, it qualified. Team CMT member Joyce Kelly helped me through the process.

Team CMT was founded in April of 2011 and we now have 78 members in 17 states. We've run dozens of events, both in the United States and Europe. I know soon we'll reach my goal of having more than 100 members. (We now have 127 members in 26 states, Canada, Iran, Turkey, Vietnam, and Australia.)

Despite hearing from several medical professionals that people with CMT shouldn't do anything too strenuous, we have 16 athletes on the team with CMT. They amaze and inspire me. This year, I'll represent Team CMT in Boston. Next year, we will have three members with qualifying times that will allow them to apply to the Boston Marathon.

I was introduced to Allison Moore of the Hereditary Neuropathy Foundation when I saw a Facebook post from her sister Kim about running the Richmond Marathon for CMT. Team CMT and HNF both share the same mission of raising awareness of CMT through athletic events. Team CMT is going to explode under the partnership with HNF. The energy Allison brings to this cause amazes me every time I talk to her. I can't wait to see her again in Boston.

I met and hired sports publicist Gail Sideman to get the word out in the media. It was Gail who arranged the TV and print media interviews. So many people now know about CMT who had never heard of it due to her efforts.

Duane Denny stepped forward to help raise money for the Boston run. Duane is a promotions professional and fitness trainer. He arranged the Boston radio interview and a fundraiser at the John Harvard Brew Pub.

I have met or emailed with athletes from all over the country. Some of them are going to be in Boston to cheer me on and come to the fundraising event. Duane Denny, Louise Gehardt, I can't wait to meet you. I am more excited about that than running the race.

Gerry Lynch was the donor matching all my Boston contributions. Gerry Lynch and his family adopted a ten-year-old girl from China last year, who has CMT. He has stepped forward to pledge $10,000 to match funds raised as part of the Boston effort. Really looking forward to meeting my large donor and his family and thanking them in person.

I'm not sure where all of this will lead or what will happen as I run the marathon. It can be a little scary to be so public about a goal. There is a big opportunity to crash and burn. So many people know about this effort and it could be embarrassing if I fail. I'm trusting that God has got me this far; He's going to get me the rest of the way.

It has been an amazing journey so far and I think it's just the beginning.

What is it that you really want to do in life? What will you commit to? Think big and be bold and then commit to it.

Chapter 58
Boston Marathon Race Eve
Unlikely Heroes

*Lord help me to do great things as though they were little,
since I do them with your power; and help me do the
little things as though they were great, since I do
them in your name.*
—Blaise Pascal, French mathematician, physicist, inventor, writer

I like biographies and stories about heroes. It is inspiring for me to hear about success against challenges and beating sometimes impossible odds.

I have two favorite heroes whom I thought about the night before the marathon.

One is Esther, found in the Bible in the book of Esther in the Old Testament. She was a young Jewish woman chosen in a sort of beauty pageant to become the new queen when the old one angered the King. She found out about a plot against her people and went before the king to plead for them at the risk of her life. Her uncle told her, "You were born for such a time as this." At a time when women were told to be seen and not heard, she found her voice. Her great risk paid off. She was able to save her people and gain the favor of the king. God had prepared her to play the part she needed to play.

I'm no beauty like Ester, but sometimes I think the many experiences I've had in my life have prepared me for this moment. Lots of things came together for me to run Boston and establish Team CMT.

Sometimes preparation comes when I am in the lowest places. I first learned that I could write when I was unemployed. I started writing training materials as an independent contractor. I had never done that and if I had not lost my job, I might never have discovered my love for and talent for writing. The low places aren't easy to go through, but they have been the times in my life when I have learned the most.

Sometimes, like Esther, I feel like I am in the right place in the right time. I, too, have found my voice— mine is to raise awareness for CMT. I will do so in Boston on one of the biggest stages possible.

The other hero who came to mind, also from the Bible, was Joseph. He was one of twelve sons of Jacob in ancient Israel. His brothers were jealous of him because he was the favorite of his father, and they sold him into slavery in Egypt. He was determined to do well despite being a slave. In his first assignment, he rose to be head of his master's household until his employer's wife falsely accused of rape He was thrown into jail and seemingly forgotten, and once again rose to a position of responsibility. When he predicted that the pharaoh's dream meant famine, he was appointed to the pharaoh's household, and soon became second in importance. Throughout his trials and tribulations, Joseph tried to do the right thing. He faced slavery, false accusations, and prison. "And the Lord was with

Joseph." Joseph was blessed in everything he did because of his faith and trust in God.

In every circumstance, God was with Joseph and He blessed everything he did. He gave Joseph gifts, which Joseph applied to succeed and rise to the top of Egyptian rulership in time to save the nation of Israel from famine.

Sometimes God finds his heroes in the most unlikely places. When God was looking for a new king in Israel, He sent his prophet to the house of Jesse. Jesse brought out his tall, strong, and handsome sons one by one. None met God's approval. The last son, the shrimp of the bunch, David, was brought forward and he was the one God wanted. David later killed the giant Goliath and became king.

So whether it's slaying giants, leading Egypt, or taking a risk to be heard, God finds a way to get His work done using the most unlikely people.

So tomorrow, while running the Boston Marathon, I will repeat those words often. The Lord was with Joseph in his challenges, and He will be with me and bless my efforts. I know I will be carrying the wishes, hopes and prayers of many friends, family members, and CMT community members.

Pictured below are some of the signatures I will carry behind my running number as I complete the Boston Marathon. I know I could not do this on my own. Yes, God does get His work done using the most unlikely people, or in this case, runner.

Tomorrow is going to be a challenging and long day. Temperatures are expected to climb to near 90F with a strong headwind. Even on a perfect day, completing a marathon is tough and challenging work.

I know I am ready physically and mentally. I can't wait for the start tomorrow, but will be even happier when—God willing—I cross the finish line.

I don't know if running Boston is a big or a little thing, but run it I will and I know I won't be doing it alone.

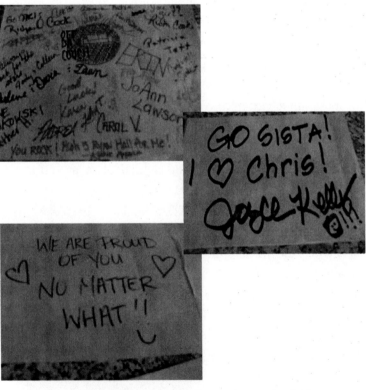

Signatures and good wishes behind my running number for Boston.

Chapter 59
Boston Marathon Dedication

What a blind person needs is not a teacher, but another self.
—Helen Keller

Because only 1 in 2,500 people have CMT, most people don't know anyone outside their immediate family with the affliction. Sometimes family members don't even talk about CMT or act as if it doesn't exist. So it's special when you find someone who both shares this condition and is an athlete as well.

I've found my "other self" in two women and will be dedicating my Boston Marathon run to them.

The first is Joyce Kelly. I wouldn't be running Boston if it weren't for Joyce. She got through to the Boston Athletic Association and found out what I had to do to apply to the Mobility Impaired Division. Joyce edited my application letter, and it was much better once she was finished with it. Joyce wanted me to get accepted to Boston as much as I did and she's been truly excited for me.

When I sent out papers to sign to attach to my running bib, Joyce sent back the signature you see pictured. She showed the same excitement when she discovered Team CMT. Joyce is also a runner and triathlete. Our experiences as athletes with

CMT are so similar, we swear we were twins separated at birth. She also makes me laugh when she tells me I'm fast.

When I visited Dallas last year, I contacted Joyce to have lunch. That was not good enough. She insisted I compete in the Denton Sprint Triathlon. She even arranged for a bike. Even though I had no plans to do the event, I qualified for the Paratriathlon National Championship in Austin. My only regret is Joyce will not be in either Boston or Austin. Injuries and life have kept Joyce from realizing her athletic dreams.

My other "sister self" is Allison Moore. Allison is president of the Hereditary Neuropathy Foundation and our Team CMT sponsor. She has provided much-needed financial and moral support for the team.

Allison was training for the New York Marathon when cancer treatments brought on the severe and immediate onset of her CMT. From the moment I first talked with Allison, I knew we shared the same goal for raising awareness about CMT through athletic events. Allison is a woman of rare vision and energy. After I talked to her on the phone, I flew to New York to meet her. I knew once I met her that it was the right move for Team CMT to join with the HNF. I felt when I talked with Allison that we'd been best friends for years.

Allison understands the significance of the Boston Marathon run. She has been with me every step of the way. When I get stressed out, she's been there to talk me off the ledge. I know she understands the drive and commitment it takes to run an event like Boston.

Allison is working hard to be able to run again. I hope the money we raise will bring us just a bit closer to making that happen. In Boston, I am running for the athletes of Team CMT and everyone struggling with this condition. Allison will be there to cheer me on, along with several other Team CMT members.

Thanks, Joyce and Allison, I will be thinking of you throughout the race and remembering the impact and influence you have had on me as an athlete.

Chapter 60

Boston Marathon—Race Day Team CMT is "All In for Boston"

*I've learned finishing a marathon isn't just an athletic
achievement. It's a state of mind; a state of mind that
says anything is possible.*
—John Hanc, author of *The Coolest Race on Earth*
and competitor in the Antarctic Marathon

Throughout the week I left for Boston, I watched the weather reports. The last one I saw said 80F on Sunday with a front moving through and temps in the 60s for race day. I remember asking a friend what would happen if the front didn't move through.

Every time I logged onto Facebook, there was another update from the B.A.A. increasing the temperature for race day. Non-elite runners were advised not to run. The final forecast was for 86F, and race day temperatures ended up being at least 89F.

I was pulled aside at the race packet pick-up by race officials. They were concerned that as a Mobility Impaired runner, I would have problems with the heat. I assured them I was well trained and would be able to handle the heat. I appreciated their care and concern. They said they would flag me in the system should I come to any first aid tent.

I felt like I'd been training for this race my whole life. Although I'd been offered a deferment because of the predicted heat, I was ready to go. I'd dedicated the run to teammates Allison Moore and Joyce Kelly. It isn't much of a dedication if you don't run. I knew if they were in my place, they would run. Lots of people were following me on Facebook and through my blog and praying for me.

I felt in my heart and soul it was the right thing to do and that I would be okay. God had gotten me this far and He wasn't going to abandon me now. I was injury free and ready to do my third marathon in a year. The Boston Marathon starts in the town of Hopkinton and winds through the small New England towns of Ashland, Natick, Wellesley, Newton and Brookline. As the signs say in every town, Team CMT was all in. It means everyone is committed. They were and so was I.

I boarded the bus on the Boston Commons at 7 am. Team CMT members Robert Kearney and Cheryl Monnat saw me off. We had all stayed together at a hotel in Cambridge right across the Charles River from Boston. I was working on about 4 1/2 hours of sleep due to a snoring roommate.

I got to the Athletes' Village at about 8 am. My wave started at 10:40 so I had lots of time to hydrate, listen to music, find some shade, and think about the race.

I was strangely calm and confident. Usually, I'm really nervous before a marathon. I've run enough of them to know the pain and fatigue that awaits me on the course. Maybe it was the signatures and good wishes written on papers I had pinned

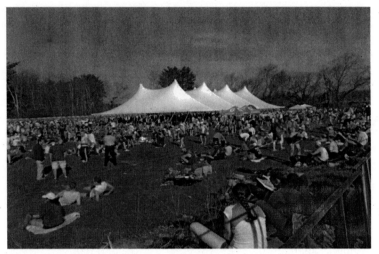

Athlete's Village- Hopkinton, Boston Marathon Start

to my numbers, maybe it was all the prayers and good wishes or the fact that I felt like I had been training for this race my whole life. I know I had trained harder for Boston than any other marathon I've ever prepared for.

I felt lucky to have gotten 4 1/2 hours of sleep the night before. I don't usually sleep at all the night before a marathon. I had worked hard I couldn't wait for the start.

Although I had banned my iPod from the race, I used it on the bus and in the Athletes' Village. Music helped to center me and mentally prepare for the day ahead.

The Boston Athletic Association has been putting on this race for over 100 years and they have everything planned. It is a major problem to get 27,000 runners started on the narrow streets of Hopkinton. To make the start go smoothly every runner is assigned a wave and a corral within the wave. Your qualification number is used to "seed" or place you in the proper start wave and corral. The faster you are the earlier you start. Elite runners are first to start. The only exceptions are the wheelchair racers and mobility impaired runners expected to take longer than six hours to finish.

There are three waves, but up to nine corrals or sections within the wave. There are about 9,000 runners in each wave. Your wave and corral are printed on the race number you must wear on race day on the front of your shirt. You line up between metal barricades on the narrow street. Signs tell you where each section or corral starts. You many move farther back in the field, but you may not move up. Volunteers monitor access into the starting area to make sure you are in the right wave and corral.

To get to the race start in Hopkinton, you must board a bus in the Boston Commons. You are assigned a time to board the bus based on your assigned wave. When you arrive in Hopkinton, you go to the athlete village which is a state park in Hopkinton. Then you wait until you are told your wave may proceed to the start. Then go to the barricade in your assigned area and a volunteer lets you in. You are packed in shoulder to shoulder with thousands of other runners, nervously waiting for the race start. It all sounds very complicated, but it all makes for a smooth and organized start on race day.

As I made my way to my corral in Wave 3, I mentally went over my plan for the day. Gone was the goal of 4:41 and even finishing in the top three in my division. I just wanted to finish. So many people were tracking me or had donated to me, I couldn't let them down. I knew on a day when the temperatures were expected to be near 90F, it would be a battle and a victory just to finish. I planned on walking a bit through every water stop.

The race started just as I got to my corral and I was off. I hit the first mile at about 9:00, way faster than I expected. I slowed down, knowing a fast pace early on would take its toll later.

My most vivid memory of this race will be the crowd support. So many families had garden hoses, buckets of water, and ice to cool down the runners. I took advantage of every one of them.

There were so many offers of orange slices, Twizzlers, pretzels, and countless other food items. Hundreds of fans stood along the course ready with cheers or high fives. Boston fans pride themselves on cheering for the last runners as much or more than the elite runners passing by early in the race. The race is a spring tradition for many locals and whole families turn out to support the runners.

The B.A.A. planned three cups of water for each runner at every water stop. I used all three: one in me and two on me. It was a struggle to try and stay cool. I carried my own sports drink so I could keep my electrolytes balanced.

I was really starting to drag at the half-way point. I was starting to doubt if I could finish. This is the tough middle of the race. Then I reached the girls of Wellesley College, who are famous for being the loudest fans on the course. They were screaming their heads off. When I yelled back, "Wellesley Girls Rock!" they screamed louder. We went back and forth and by the time I was past them, I was ready to rock and roll. I felt great!

I've never had support on the course when I've run a marathon before. So it was a real treat to have Cheryl Monnat waiting at mile 17. I think I looked pretty good although I was struggling. I had so much water in my shoes it was sloshing around. Time for a quick stop for dry shoes and socks. I also got a full bottle of sports drink and GU. I was off and then met Allison Moore and friend Valarie at mile 21. Stop for a quick picture, hug, and encouragement. By the time I hit Mile 20, I knew I going to finish. I was splitting my time between walking and running. Almost everyone was—we all looked like the walking wounded.

I saw runners down and lots in the first aid tents. One runner collapsed in the last .2 miles. Imagine getting that far and not be able to finish.

It was no time at all before I was headed down Boylston Street lined with thousands of cheering fans and the finish line. I don't know how she did it, but Cheryl was at Mile 25 as well. I cannot tell you how much the support helped. I came down Boylston lined with a sea of people, all cheering like I was the first runner they were seeing.

Running through the tunnel of fans to the finish is an experience I will never forget. I was even hydrated enough to shed a few tears. Running Boston has been an emotional experience I will never forget.

I was so excited and happy to finish!

Now all I had to do was get my finisher medal, pick up luggage, and meet Cheryl. While I waited, I propped my feet up against a building wall. I got a couple of killer leg cramps, so I think I had finished just in time. My time was a terrible 5:27, but I finished. I am a little disappointed in my time. I ran safe, but not the great race I am capable of running.

Could I have gone faster? Maybe. But it didn't seem worth the risk. As an athlete, I have to listen to my body. That a day saw 252 runners go to the hospital and 2,000 treated on the course. I chose to be conservative and finish.

I not only finished, I took 2nd in the Mobility Impaired Division. If I had pushed it a bit more, I could have had 1st.

I guess I just have something to look forward to next year. Running a marathon is more than just conquering the distance. It's also about mastering your mind to let your body do the things it's meant to do. Sometimes the biggest limits we have are the ones we set on ourselves. That happened a bit during this race. I know I still have a ways to go to fully push myself in a marathon. Can't wait till the next one.

Team CMT member Trenni finished in 4 hours 5 minutes. Way to go, Trenni!!

I was not the only one that struggled. My elite runner ex was 40 minutes slower than usual. Last year's top men's and women's runners did not finish. All in all, it was a good day— one I will always remember.

Chapter 61

Boston Marathon
Fenway Post-Party

Pain is temporary, quitting lasts forever.
—Lance Armstrong

I don't know if Lance said that before or after he ran the New York Marathon. Anyone who's run a marathon knows the legs can feel it for a few days. No matter. I finished! It was time to hit the marathon post marthon party at Fenway Park. Cheryl had never been there so we had to go. Fenway park built in 1912 is the oldest baseball stadium in America still in use It is built within the city of Boston so it is one of the smallest parks there is no parking. It is famous for quirks like the Green Monster, the 37 foot 2 inch high left field wall. Fenway has a charm all its own. It can be a tough ticket to get since the stadium holds the record for most consecutive sell outs at 794 regular season games and 820 with the post season. It should be on any baseball fan's must see list.

There were 27,000 runners in town for the marathon and standing right in the entrance to Fenway was my ex-boyfriend, the elite runner.

Of all the places in Boston he happened to be there right in the only open gate. He was wearing his finisher medal and I thought what a geek. His race had been over hours ago. No one wears their finisher medal after the race. His fiancé was not there so just who was he trying to impress? At that moment, I knew I was over him and glad he was out of my life.

Cheryl and I ignored him and took a look at the field. We checked out the inside of the stadium and listened to the music for a few minutes. Since I did not want to run into my ex, we only stayed a few minutes. Totally missed getting our picture taken of the World Series trophies.

I walked right past him on the way out, standing by himself still wearing his finisher medal. Maybe he was waiting for friends to go to the other after-party at the House of Blues. Loud music and crowds were not my idea of a good time after spending 5½ hours on my feet in brutally hot weather.

It was still in the 80's even after dark. The only hot weather clothes I had were a Boston Marathon T-shirt and a running skirt I bought at the expo. It seemed okay since everyone at Fenway seemed to be runners since many were wearing shirts from runs in other cities.

I had not eaten much all day and was really getting hungry. Since all they had was ball park food at Fenway, we needed to be on our way. We stopped for a few photos at the Teammates statue outside of Fenway. Some guy wanted his photo taken with me. We actually match. Guess we're a couple.

I needed food, not booze. I had been drinking water for hours after the race and was not sweating anything out. I was a bit worried and didn't think alcohol was a good idea. Cheryl and I instead headed to an Italian area for pizza and pasta. Robert was not able to join us since he left earlier in the day for a business trip to Germany. He joined Cheryl on the course for a bit to watch the runners and then caught the train to the airport to catch his flight.

We were home by 10 p.m. for some well-deserved rest. I can't wait to come back and run again next year and spend a little more time at the post-marathon party. Hopefully I won't run into any former friends again.

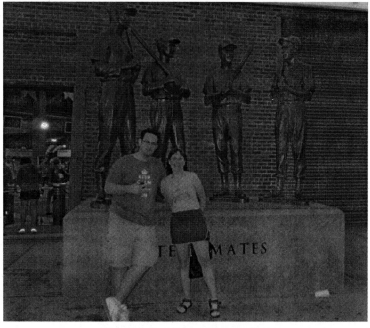

Marathon Post-Party at Fenway Park

Chapter 62
Boston's Done! What's Next?

The finish line is just the beginning of a whole new race.
—Unknown

There was a reason I was so calm and cool about the Boston Marathon. I knew I had another event following closely after. I stayed calm in Boston by focusing on all the things I needed to do to get ready for my next event.

On May 28th, 2012, I was going to participate in the USA Paratriathlon National Championship in Austin, Texas. With only 6 weeks between events, after I got home to Milwaukee, I went right into training for the tri. I was really supposed to be in recovery mode. It takes about a day to recover for every mile you run. That meant I should be taking a bit easy for 26 days or so, not training for another event, much less a national championship.

The athlete finishing first in each category will represent the USA at the World Championships in Auckland, New Zealand in October. I am still trying to wrap my mind around the fact that I am going to a national competition with a shot at becoming a member of the U.S. team. It was a chance I couldn't pass up.

I never expected to be running such an event this soon. Last year, just for fun, I ran the Denton Pioneer Sprint

Triathlon. I did about a month's worth of swim training and a bit of biking, since I was already training for Marine Corps Marathon. To my surprise, my performance was good enough to land me a qualifying spot. So National Championship, ready or not, here I come.

I started to get nervous every time I thought about the nationals, so running Boston seemed like no big deal. It was marathon number seven, after all. I feel like I have been running and racing half my adult life. It seems second nature now and I know just what to do. The Championship will be triathlon number five, so I am still a novice.

Making lists helps me combat my fears and getting everything ready helps me to fight my nerves. I know the swim will be tough, since I am not experienced at open water swims. I got a little practice at a recent swim clinic and was shown some good techniques for turning around the buoy.

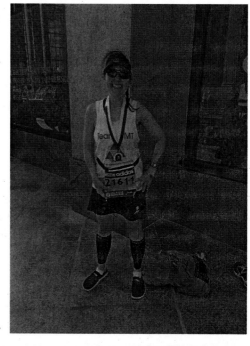

Boston 2012 done.

Chapter 63
Obsession

Obsessed is just a word the lazy use to describe the dedicated.
— Unknown

Just ten days to go until the National Sprint Championship in Austin Texas. I know I like to compete and work out, but I didn't realize until this week just what an obsession they are. I've been thrown yet another challenge as I get ready for Austin.

I have been fighting an injury on my right ankle. It happened right after a swim clinic about 3 weeks after Boston. I remember bumping my ankle at work and finding the pea-sized knot on my ankle. It hurt like hell. At first I thought it was tendonitis, which could have sidelined me for weeks, since that takes a long time to heal.

It's probably the result of running three marathons in the last year, including the very hot and hilly Boston Marathon just over a month ago. I went right from Boston into training for Nationals. Maybe I was trying to do just a little too much.

It seems to be a muscle knot and it is putting a serious crimp in my training plans. To have a shot at the national championship I am going to have to run my absolute best race. I can't do that if I'm injured. If I stop training to let it heal, I lose valuable time for the physical and mental preparation.

With running, I can usually work around most minor injuries. So I tried to keep training and it didn't really work.

First I stopped running except in the pool. I kept up with the cycling, including a hilly two-hour ride on a date in Governor Dodge Park in western Wisconsin. The pain in my ankle got so bad that I took two days off in a row, which I don't even do when I'm sick.

One day, when it hurt to drive, I knew I had to take drastic measures. So I may be taking I stopped running for four days off to see if I could get my ankle to heal. I haven't had that many days off since I had shoulder surgery 14 years ago. It is drove me crazy. Working out is such a part of my routine it just doesn't feel right not to be doing something. Most days, I train in at least two and sometimes three sports. I love it and really miss working out when I can't.

The injury takes a mental toll as well. I always question if I've done enough of the right training for an event. Now I will have to second-guess both the decision to keep working out and now to take time off. My coach and doctor both assure me my performance won't suffer much. I guess we will find out race day. I know I would feel more mentally prepared if I were working hard. Doing nothing is harder for me than working out. I can't wait until I can bike, swim, and run pain free. I love being active and miss it. I get some of my best ideas when running. I can't even remember the last time I ran.

So, yes, I am probably obsessed, but I think it's a pretty healthy obsession. Let's hope the rest helps and that I can resist the temptation to start exercising before I'm healed.

Chapter 64
Good Enough for Boston, But Not for Austin

You miss 100% of the shots you never take.
—Wayne Gretzke, hockey player

n April, I was accepted to run in the Mobility Impaired Division of the Boston Marathon based on my diagnosis of CMT.

Paratriathlon is a variant of the triathlon for athletes with a physical disability. Paratriathlon includes a sprint distance event with a 750m swim, 20K cycling using handcycles, bicycles, tricycles, or tandem bicycles with a guide, and a 5Kwheelchair or running race. Athletes compete in six categories according to the nature of their physical impairments.

Before being allowed to compete at the Paratriathlon National Championship, I had to be assessed. There is one assessor in the entire country, who makes the decision if you meet the criteria to compete. There are six categories in Paratriathlon competition, of which I was hoping to qualify for TRI 3, because CMT falls under Muscular Dystrophy. According to the USA Triathlon (USAT):

TRI 3, known as *Les Autres* or "the Others": Includes athletes with Multiple Sclerosis, Muscular Dystrophy, Cerebral Palsy, Double Leg Amputee (runners) or Paralysis in multiple limbs. Must have a minimum of 15% impairment of any one limb. Must ride a bicycle or tricycle and run. May use cane, braces or prosthesis during run portion. No racing wheelchairs.

Minimum Disability Standard
A specific "Minimum Disability Standard" is also enforced. We know that this may have a significant impact on many athletes (especially in the "Les Autres" category) so please read them very carefully:

An athlete has to show a15% impairment in any one limb to qualify in TRI 3. Each athlete is assessed for placement in the appropriate category based on their impairment. This is to have athletes with similar impairments competing against each other. Paratriathlon has been accepted as a Para-Olympic sport starting in 2016.

The top finisher in each division would win a spot on the national team and a chance to compete in the World Championship.

USA Triathlon (USAT) is the national governing body for the multisport disciplines of triathlon, dualthon, aquathon, and winter triathlon in the United States. USA Triathlon is a member federation of the U.S. Olympic Committee and the International Triathlon Union (ITU).

There is usually only one chance for assessment per year in the United States. That opportunity happens at the National Championship events, and this year, it was in Austin. I talked with the Paratriathlon manager for USAT to determine the assessment criteria. She would not tell me and could not discuss how I would be assessed or what would be measured. I could not travel anywhere to meet an assessor before the competition. There was one trained assessor in the United States and she would assess in Austin.

The process is very secret and at least for me, not very extensive. I knew there was a pretty good chance after the time, expense, and preparation that I might not be allowed into the National Championship.

Once in Austin, I submitted notes from the neurology exam that had gotten me into the Boston Marathon. After a few questions about how CMT affects my swimming, biking, and running, the physical therapist present did a few strength and range of motion tests.

The strength test consisted of me pushing against her resistance. A child could have pushed harder. It was completely ridiculous. Right from the start, I could tell they did not take my CMT seriously.

I have been examined by four neurologists and many physical therapists. The assessor used the same strength and balance tests as these medical professionals. However, the difference was the amount of force used by the USAT assessor. No pressure at all was used and I do not think it was an accurate test. In fact, it was a complete farce. It did not measure my impairment at all.

The assessor did not even measure the flexibility in my ankles, which is one of my most severe impairments. She tried to flex my ankle, then just called out the number to an assistant. I can flex my ankle backward less than half of a normal person. That is because my calf muscles and tendons are so tight due to the CMT. I don't have enough flexibility to walk normally, much less swim, run, and bike. It is a major limiting factor in my athletic ability and she did not even measure it.

After mere minutes, the assessment was over. I was told I was not "impaired enough" and "too strong." Dee (not her real name), the woman who started the CMTA Athletes team, was also rejected. I thought it would be awkward seeing her after her negative posts and returning her Team CMT kit. She had contacted me by email before the assessment, offering to put together my bike. I thought that was nice and was willing to extend my friendship. After we both failed our assessment, we spent some time talking about the experience and sharing our disappointment.

It didn't matter to the USAT assessor that the Boston Marathon accepted my CMT or that the International Triathlon Union has given me the provisional classification I was seeking based on a review of my medical records. Now that I have gone through USA Triathlon (USAT) process, the ITU classification was no longer valid.

I feel the strength alone measurement is not fair, since I have worked hard to preserve both strength and function. I would like the USAT officials to see the bills for chiropractic care, physical therapy, massages, and doctor care. It is a struggle every day to maintain the activity level necessary to try and compete on any level.

It was not a surprise to be rejected, since CMT is not well understood even in the medical community. Ignorance about CMT is something we face every day. How disappointing to see it once again at the national level.

However, I could compete in the open division and represent Team CMT. The open division was for athletes who could not meet the time standard or classify into the race.

USAT promised to take a look at the classification process for TRI 3 for 2013. I can only hope they are open to education about CMT and its effect on athletes. The mission of Team CMT has been to raise awareness and educate. I just didn't think I would need to educate the USAT.

Chapter 65
My Own Worst Enemy

It is not the mountains we conquer, but ourselves.
—Sir Edmund Hilary, climber of Mt. Everest

Sir Edmund could have been talking about me as I raced the Cap Tex Tri. Physically Challenged Open Division at the National Paratriathlon Sprint Championship. I was my own worst enemy. Inexperience, mistakes, and disappointment were all demons against which I battled.

It all started the day I did not classify into the TRI3 Paratriathlete category. I was told I was not impaired enough and too strong. Gone was any shot at the National Championship and a chance to compete at the World Championships. I was transferred into the physically challenged open division, which meant I had to give back the number with my name and national championship designation. That hurt, for it meant I could complete, but not have a chance at being on Team USA and to go to the Paratriathlon World Championship in Auckland, New Zealand.

Later in the day, when I took out the rental bike for a test ride, the tire was flat and had to be taken back to the shop. I rented a bike because I did not want to deal with the hassle of traveling on an airplane with a bike. To get my bike to Austin, it would have to be taken apart, packed in a bike carrier bag, and then taken to a shop to put back together for the race. The whole process would have to be repeated for the trip home. I only got to do a short test ride on the rental bike since members of my family were waiting for me.

The race would be a ¼ mile swim, 12-mile bike ride and 3.1-mile run. The swim was in Lady Bird Lake near the Texas state capitol building. The bike course consisted of two loops in the area around the Capitol and the University of Texas. The run was a rather unscenic route along city streets.

On race day, I was denied access to the transition area. I had racked my bike in the sprint area according to the number I had been assigned. I did not know there was a rack in a different area for those competing in the paratriathlon championship wave and open division. It seemed like it took forever to get a race official over and get me to the right transition area. I felt like I barely had time to set up my gear and that added to my stress.

I also had trouble getting into the swim start until I pointed out to the official I had the same color swim cap as the athletes in the water. Once in the water, my goggles fogged despite the defog goop I had applied. Then, even though I rinsed the goggles, the defog stung my eyes. As I looked at the triangular course at the buoys in the open water, the swim looked so far. I had to remind myself I had been swimming twice that distance in practice.

When you can count on one hand the number of triathlons you have done, you're not a pro. I had only done five, four of which had open-water swims. My lack of experience showed in the swim. The course we were to swim was triangular. I had seen the map and had it explained to me. The swim was going fine. I made my fancy turn around the buoy like I had learned at swim clinic. The only problem was it was the wrong turn. I was asked by one of the race marshals if I was okay and was then informed I had missed the turn. I had to go back and redo it. Still, I did the crawl stroke the entire way, which was a big improvement over previous races.

During the bike leg, my race belt must have come undone and I lost my number. I informed the race official in transition about what happened and was instructed to complete the course. I was scored, but if I had been in the National Championship, that mistake would have gotten me disqualified. I also missed a turn around on the bike leg. Even though I did not miss by much, it cost me some time. I also hugged the right side of the course to stay out of the way of all the elite athletes speeding by me. The run was the only part of the race that went smoothly, since biking is also where I have the most experience.

I was also racing without a bike computer since the rental bike did not have one, which I had not noticed until the flat was fixed. So I was basically racing blind. I wouldn't know my speed until race results were published.

Well, I have a lot to learn and a lot of mistakes to correct for next time. My clock time when I crossed the finish line was 1 hour 45 minutes. I would have known my time if I had remembered to start the watch I was wearing. Chip times have been published and I finished just a bit over 1 hour and 39 minutes.

Every athlete is given a timing chip to wear around their left ankle. It looks like a Velcro strap, but has a plastic chip programmed with the athlete's number. It tracks swim time, bike time, run time, and times spent transitioning between swim and bike and bike and run.

I raced like a complete moron, but still managed to win the Physically Challenged Open Division. I even beat the time of the winner in TRI 3, the category in which I was denied entry. I am looking forward to the next time and maybe, just maybe, a spot in the National Championship race.

If I had classified, I would have been National Champion, at least based on the times published on race day. Those times and finish would soon come into question.

Chapter 66

Championship Won, Championship Lost

*Our lives begin to end the day we become silent
about things that matter.*
—Dr. Martin Luther King, Jr.

When I moved my bike from one transition area to another on race day, I lost track of my family. My brother Tony and his wife had driven down from Dallas with me. We had planned on picking a meeting place, but got separated when I moved to the other transition area where the paratriathletes were. Because I did not have a cell phone with me, I was not able to find out where they were. My brother had planned on handing me his cell phone, but that fell through. It took so long to let me into the original transition area, I barely had time to get ready and be at the start line.

The Cap Tex Triathlon is a huge race with around 3,000 participants. It took two hours of wandering around in the heat before I was able to find my family after the race. I borrowed a cell phone from someone in the park and left a message at their house, hoping one of the kids would pick up the message and call my sister's cell phone. Then I went to the bike shop where I had rented the bike. I left messages with two of my brothers, asking them to call and try and get in touch with one of my nephews so they NOT Sure what you wanted to put here.

Because I had been so focused on finding my sister and nephews, I had no idea when the awards were presented. I did not know I had won the Open Division until I got back to Dallas that afternoon and checked the results on the Internet. I had also beaten the time of the TRI 3 champion, the division I had hoped to get into, by about a dozen seconds. Considering all the mistakes I made, I was happy with the outcome—I was National Champion of the Open Division.

Someone this week complimented me on how positive I am and how she wishes her husband could be more like me.

The news I got later that week made it impossible to maintain my positive attitude. I was angry about some things that happened during the Cap Tex Tri, both before, after, and during the race.

When I entered, I thought it would be a great opportunity to raise awareness and educate about CMT. I had spent a great deal of time and money getting ready for Austin. As I mentioned above, after a very brief exam, I was pronounced not "impaired" enough and too strong. The assessor never looked at the detailed medical notes provided by one of my doctors. Although disappointed, I had not expected to classify in. Most medical professionals do not know much about CMT and I looked forward to helping the USAT better understand CMT and its effect on athletes.

My intention was to compete in the Physically Challenged Open Division, in which I would be competing against athletes who faced similar impairments. The National

Championship wave was for the athletes who passed the medical classification. The Open Division was for the athletes who were not fast enough to qualify for the Championship wave or did not pass the classification process.

Dee, the American triathlete living in England, was also in Austin. I looked forward to being in the same race. It was fantastic to meet her and get to know her. Dee had not classified into the TRI 3 National Championship wave. A bit of competition exists between us since she started CMT Athletes after leaving Team CMT. On race day, we both lined up in the Open Division.

I competed, made lots of mistakes, but still managed to finish first in the Open Division. Or so I thought. The USAT website had posted a story about the Paratriathlon events and listed me as the Women's winner in the Open Division. When I checked the listing prior to posting the link on my own website, another woman had been listed as the Open Division winner!

Immediately, I sent an email off to the USAT to ask about the change. My email was sent to the Cap Tex Tri race director. After several emails, I discovered what happened.

An athlete in TRI6 (visual impairment) had raced for the National Championship and placed 4th. A nice day and my congratulations to her. What happened next is where I have an issue.

The athlete decided she also wanted to compete in the Open Division. Because our waves were consecutive, it was not possible for her to start in the Open Division wave. She was allowed to line up with the age-group athletes and was scored against those of us in the Open Division. She raced twice and was awarded two places.

At the very least, that was a major violation of USAT rules. The rules state if you don't start in your assigned wave, you are not eligible for awards. In my opinion, it was also bad sportsmanship on the part of the athlete to claim two awards— and a bad decision on the part of race officials to make this decision. It is even worse to stick to that decision when it is brought to your attention.

As a visually impaired athlete, the woman races on a tandem bike and has the assistance of an able-bodied partner. By no means do I wish to downplay her impairment or her accomplishment. She had that chance when she qualified for and raced in the National Championship wave. Racing against those of us with CMT is not a fair match. That is why there are six categories in the paratriathlon races. It is also not fair to be able to race twice.

This isn't golf; you don't get a mulligan. You don't get to keep racing until you like the result. I was told the race officials made an exception. So what that she did the course twice. What is the big deal?

It isn't only the fact I was knocked into 2nd place. I am used to finishing well back in the pack. For once in my life, it had been a chance to compete on a level playing field. After not getting into the National Championship wave, it was the only event I had left. I felt discounted as an athlete when the USAT and race officials causally let someone into the category who had already competed. It was a tough pill to swallow after the superficial assessment of my CMT I was given by the assessor. The woman still has a chance to be on the U.S. team and go to the World Championships in New Zealand. So why enter the only competition open to those of us who were in the Open Division?

What was even more upsetting is that neither the USAT or race officials could understand why this was a problem. I cried as I wrote my reply to them because they so clearly did not understand the daily struggles faced by anyone with CMT, athlete or not. Those of us with CMT are challenged by the effects of CMT, and secondly by ignorance about the very existence of the disease.

I have been called a scammer because I want to compete in events like the Boston Marathon or the Nationals. I've learned to expect ignorance and arrogance from uneducated members of the public. However, I never expected to find such attitudes in race officials or in the USAT, particularly when visually or physically impaired athletes are involved. I was made to feel like a fraud all over again. I would like any athlete, race official, or USAT officer to run a race in my shoes.

I would give anything to be a normal athlete. It is so hard to watch CMT steal my ability bit by bit and know there is nothing I can do about it. Being moved to second place totally dismisses the realities faced by any of us with CMT.

So I couldn't stay silent. I feel like I speak for everyone living and struggling with CMT. I felt compelled to make my case even if no one understands why or how important it is. It is a struggle for acceptance and recognition.

Perhaps it's difficult for anyone reading this to understand why I am upset. I know I should be happy I can still run and compete. The possibility of competing at a national level has been a major motivation. When I was tired and didn't want to work out, I would remind myself my competitors were working out.

At this point, I am so completely discouraged that I have even thought about not doing another triathlon. There is one on my schedule, but it is a USAT-sanctioned event. I'm not sure if I will go. I am not excited about it at all, but if I don't go, I may never do another triathlon again. If I stop competing, I may stop working out. If I don't work out, my CMT will progress more quickly and I will be the real loser.

The Cap Tex Tri was so exhausting, I could barely function the following week. So maybe things that would normally not bother me really got to me. That is also part of being an athlete with CMT. Events like this in the heat are exhausting. For race officials to so causally allow in someone who had already competed is discouraging beyond words.

Am I being overly dramatic and emotional? Maybe, but heart and emotion are what fuel me as an athlete. I wouldn't be able to get my body to do the things I do without them. Right now, I can't summon either energy or emotion. This race and my interaction with the race director have drained me. I felt like no one understood and no one cared.

Chapter 67
CMT and the Butterfly Effect

I do not sing because I am happy, I am happy because I sing.
—Unknown

Have you ever heard the term "butterfly effect"? The phrase refers to the idea that a butterfly's wings might create tiny changes in the atmosphere that may ultimately alter the path of a tornado or delay, accelerate, or even prevent the occurrence of a tornado in another location.

Andy Andrews, in his book *The Butterfly Effect*, talks about how some simple acts have profoundly changed history. He contends the simplest acts you do can have great impact and meaning. He draws the connections between simple acts and great events in history. Like Andrews, I like to see the connections.

Team CMT member 100 caused her own butterfly effect. I had asked my niece to become a member of Team CMT because it would not exist without her.

About three years ago, she went to her foot doctor because she was falling and breaking bones in her feet. Her doctor called in every favor he had to get her tested at Children's Hospital in Philadelphia. Genetic testing confirmed that she had Charcot-Marie-Tooth type 1a. If you had seen her feet, you would have known right away—she has the high arches and hammer toes characteristic of CMT. The little toes on her feet stick straight up. When her mom emailed me about the CMT, I was curious and did my own Google search. When I read the list of symptoms, I knew I had CMT as well and got my own diagnosis in August of 2010.

I had never heard of CMT and it just did not seem right to me that I had a disease no one had ever heard of. I was also surprised at the reluctance of my own family to talk about a condition many of us share.

I knew I was really lucky to still be running, so I decided to use that gift to raise awareness about this potentially debilitating disease. Team CMT was born from my experience with running races to raise awareness about other illnesses.

I often think about the person who gave the gift to Philadelphia Children's Hospital that allowed my niece to get her genetic test. The anonymous donor could not have known about the profound effect his or her simple gift has had. After my niece was diagnosed with CMT, I was able to get my answers as well.

We can all make a difference and we all have a purpose in our lives. Sometimes we do not know what kind of a difference we can make or see the impacts of our actions, but they are there.

When I think back about my niece as a baby and little girl, I remember her as someone who was always smiling, laughing, and talking. I can see why the foot doctor went the extra mile for her.

To her, CMT is no "biggie" and she refuses to let it change her. She recently turned 18 and is off to study marine biology at college. She may have CMT, but it does not have her. Even though she can't run or bike, she has maintained her sunny and happy disposition.

I have not used my niece's name here because she has chosen to keep her CMT a secret. While she gladly accepted the offer to be on Team CMT, she has not wanted to publically acknowledge her membership.

I can understand that. She's in her first year of college, a time in which friends' opinions matter. She is trying to date and figure out what to do with the rest of her life. To her, explaining about her CMT is just too complicated in an already too-busy life.

Her family is like many with CMT, who struggle in silence, thinking that their CMT is no big deal, or they suffer in silence, afraid of what others might think or how they will act.

Those of us with CMT have nothing to be ashamed of. We didn't do anything to get CMT. We didn't eat the wrong foods or share IV needles or anything else to "get" CMT. The simple act of being born gave us CMT. We did not choose to have CMT, but we can choose what we do about it.

We can choose to do nothing and continue to let CMT be a disease no one has ever heard of, or we can acknowledge our condition in hopes of making a difference. Every person willing to step forward creates his or her own "butterfly effect."

So, while running events, wearing Team CMT gear, and blogging may seem like small things, they are having a big effect. Team CMT is creating its own butterfly effect. Every CMT-affected athlete on this team has made the choice to step forward and be public about this condition. These members are leading the way for others to talk about their own CMT. I hope our efforts are a source of pride for the CMT community. I know we are showing others that they can be active and lead a full life with CMT.

Who would have thought a simple doctor's appointment could have led to this.

I know our simple acts to raise awareness making a huge difference. I can't wait to see what effects Team CMT will have in the future.

So next time you see a butterfly, think about my niece, Team CMT, all of us with CMT, and how simple acts can have profound effects.

Chapter 68
Championship Regained

More often in life, we end up regretting the chances
in life we had, but didn't take, than those chances we took
and wish we hadn't.
—Unknown

When the race result changed for the Austin Championship, I tried to resolve the issue with the race director and with USAT's paratriathlon manager. I got nowhere. The race director kept saying it was his decision to score a racer in first place in my division, even though the racer had not started with the Open Division wave.

USAT has lots or rules the participants must follow. I quoted to the race director the rule that the race participant must start with one wave to be scored in that wave. He would not budge in his decision. He was the race director, it was his decision, and he was sticking to it.

When I told my coach what was going on, she got on the phone to USAT headquarters in Colorado Springs. She talked with the Commissioner of Officials, who told us to file an appeal.

What we did not know at the time was that he was in Austin because the Cap Tex Tri was a National Championship race. All rule changes and requests had to be okayed by him.

The race director never talked about letting a race participant be in two waves in the same race and did not give an exemption from the rules.

It took a couple of tries, but I got the appeal form and sent it with my check for $100, the fee for filing the appeal, to USAT.

Then I waited. After what seemed like forever, a hearing was scheduled. I was not required to attend the phone conference, but would be allowed to state my case. My coach, the race director, and the athlete involved were all invited.

What made things a bit awkward for me was I had had email contact with the other athlete. I had written a blog about what happened. I said I thought it was poor sportsmanship on the part of the other athlete. She had qualified for the National Championship wave in the visually impaired division. She finished fourth. Then she lined up with the age group wave hours later and asked to be scored in the Open Division wave, in which I had raced.

As a visually impaired athlete, she has a guide. The pair rides a tandem during the bike portion of the race. Of course, with her impairment, she needs a guide. I just thought it was an unfair advantage for a solo biker to have to race against a tandem. Tandem bikes are much faster and it is hard for an athlete like me with compromised legs to beat a tandem.

I felt she had her shot at a National Championship and a chance to be on the U.S. team. The Open Division was for those athletes who did not or could not qualify for the Championship wave. Some could not meet the time standard. Others, like me, were not allowed in.

To me, it felt like a bit of a medal grab. Dee, the other CMT-affected athlete who raced in the Open Division sent the link of the blog to the other athlete. Her response: an email saying she raced in the two divisions because she was training for an Iron Man competition and maybe I should train harder next time.

Needless to say, I was not looking forward to being on the same conference call with the athlete or with the race director. As the email exchange went on, I will admit things got contentious on my side. I was not exactly proud of how angry I was, so I was not looking forward to another encounter with the race director either.

I know I had not done anything wrong, but I still felt like I was on trial. I was one of the first to join the phone conference, followed by my coach Joy Von Werder, the Commissioner of Officials for USAT, and three panel members—all lawyers. It was all a bit intimidating and I was really glad to have Joy in my corner. Neither the race director nor the other athlete joined the phone conference for the hearing.

I actually did not have to say much. The Commissioner of Officials spoke about how USAT was in the unusual position of agreeing with my appeal. The facts were read out from my appeal form. Joy made a brief statement, and I had to answer a few questions. The lawyers on the panel asked lots of questions. It all seemed really silly and I think they were a bit incredulous about what had happened.

It was all over fairly quickly. The conference closed with a statement saying the group would deliberate and I should have a decision within a month. Following is a portion of the letter I got about three weeks later with the decision. I have replaced the name of the athlete involved.

Facts and Background

The facts of this matter are not in dispute. The Capital of Texas Triathlon in Austin, Texas was selected to serve as the USA Triathlon Paratriathlon National Championship. Paratriathletes from across the country competed there for national titles and spots on Team USA for the Paratriathlon World Championship. Participants for the Paratriathlon National Championship Division were required to be formally classified as eligible to compete in the category appropriate to the participant's disability. USA Triathlon, in order to accommodate disabled athletes who fail to classify in a specific category, or who are unable or unwilling to follow the strict rules of Paratriathlon, has created a division called PC Open. Athletes who traveled to Austin for the event and who were not classified as TRI 1, TRI 2, TRI 3, TRI 4, TRI 5, or TRI 6, were placed in the PC Open Division.

The Paratriathlon National Championship Division had a start time of 7:00 a.m. The PC Open Division had a start time of 7:10 a.m. A Sprint Category for the Age Group division of the Triathlon began at 9:10 a.m. Appellant had hoped to classify as a TRI 3 in Austin; however, the classification team made a determination that she did not meet the minimum disability standard to place her in that category. Accordingly, she was placed in the PC Open Division. Though disappointed, she committed to racing and hoped to be the best in her category. USA Triathlon sent the Commissioner of Officials to the event because of the importance of National Championships to the sport. The Commissioner has the most experience of any official with Paratriathlon and he reached out to race management several months before the event to offer his guidance with respect to any question of the rules. He asked that any issues or questions about the legality of equipment or behavior be directed to him for a ruling. The Commissioner gave the pre-race rules briefing for both Paratriathletes and PC Open participants.

At some point prior to the event, race management made an arrangement with a TRI 6 participant, to allow her to compete in two divisions, once as a properly classified TRI 6 in the Paratriathlon National Championship division and also in the PC Open Division.

The Triathlon took place on May 28, 2012. T6 actually competed in the Paratriathlon National Championship (Tri 6) division beginning with the TRI 6 wave and again in a Sprint Wave with a start time of 9:10 a.m. It is undisputed that TRI6 athlete did not start with the PC Open Division at 7:10 a.m.

TRI6 athlete although she did not start with the PC Open Division, was declared the PC Open Division national champion based on the time she achieved when she began at 9:10 a.m. with the Sprint Wave participants. Appellant, although her time was faster than all other competitors who began with the PC Open Division, was declared the second place finisher.

Decision
Based on the evidence provided by Appellant in her Petition of Appeal, the Position of USA Triathlon Regarding the Christine

Wodke Appeal and additional submissions by USAT, the testimony provided by Appellant, and the testimony of the Commissioner of Officials, Appellant's appeal is GRANTED.

Participants are required to start with their wave or group or they will not be eligible for awards in that group. The relevant portion of Article 3.4m Wave Starts states:

Wave Starts. When the beginning of any event is commenced by starting designated "waves" or groups of participants at different times, all participants shall start in and with the proper wave or group. Any request for a variance from USA Triathlon rules and policies must be done according to Article 1.4 of the Competitive Rules:

1.4 Rules Exceptions and Additions. For any particular event, a race director may request from USA Triathlon a specific exception or addition to these Rules. Any such request should be made with the consideration of the participant's safety as the highest priority. All requests for Rule changes must be made in writing. All exceptions or additions to these Rules must be expressly approved in writing by the Executive Director of USA Triathlon and must be announced to all participants prior to the event.

The wave start time for the PC Open Division for the Triathlon was 7:10 a.m. TRI6 athlete did not begin at the start time. The Race Director did not request an exception to the start time for TRI6 athlete prior to the race. The USAT Commissioner of Officials was present at the race and readily accessible to consider any request. Accordingly, any decision to use a start time of 9:10 a.m. to record the time of TRI6 athlete for the PC

Open Division does not accord with the USAT Competitive
Rules. The time recorded for TRI6 athlete for the PC Open
Division was erroneous. The Panel GRANTS the appeal of
Appellant. TRI6 athlete is disqualified from the PC Open
Division of the Capital of Texas Triathlon held on May 28, 2012.
Accordingly, Ms. Wodke is the first place finisher and national
champion in the PC Open Division of the USA Triathlon
Paratriathlon National Championship held at the Capital of
Texas Triathlon on May 28, 2012."

Even after the decision, my battle with the race director was not over. I wanted and deserved my first-place finisher medal. I sent repeated email requests, which were ignored. I again had to enlist the help of USAT. About a month after I got the decision, I received my first-place medal in the mail. The race director pointed out to me I had not won a National Championship. I pointed him to the decision that stated I was indeed the National Champion of the Open Division.

This was exactly the same lack of respect he had shown to me as an athlete in all of his previous emails. It was one of the reasons I filed the appeal. The USAT stood behind me as an athlete and I am grateful. The race director is a former USAT president, so the organization could easily have ignored my request. I was so grateful that someone listened and cared about what happened. I was later told my case would be used in the future to train race directors and officials.

Chapter 69
Time Between the Lines

I need something—the distraction of another life—
to alleviate fear.
—Bret Easton Ellis, American author

I've heard professional athletes say they leave behind their problems during the time they are on the field. That time between the lines is when trouble fades and there is only the game or the race. In a fall triathon, I needed my own time between the lines.

As I stood at on the beach waiting for the start of the TriRock Triathlon on September of 2012, I honestly did not want to be there. It had nothing to do with the 34-degree temperature or the 6:30 a.m. start. I'd been competing since May with a muscle knot on my ankle and it was getting worse. Staying home would have been smart. But I had told Team CMT member Kevin Klein I would be there. The last time we were in the same race was at Pleasant Prairie, Wisconsin, in June and I bailed from exhaustion in the swim. I needed to redeem myself.

I honestly had almost given up participating in triathlons. I blew off doing several triathlons this summer because mentally I just didn't feel like it.

My previous bad experience at Pleasant Prairie did not help. But I bounced back with two really good races at Portage and Fredonia and again qualified for Nationals the next May in Austin. I was back and excited about competing again.

* * * * *

Then life intervened and I found my mind far away as I stood waiting for the start. My 81-year-old dad recently entered the hospital and a nursing home. He was three hours away, and I wanted to be with him. Right after the race, I would be driving there.

When my dad entered the hospital, my youngest brother had the responsibility of managing his finances. My brother soon found out my dad had virtually no money. Only a year ago, Dad had a healthy savings account balance. We discovered that all his money had gone to his-ex girl friend and her daughter. We think the amount was at least $71,000, or maybe more. My dad has dementia, making him an easy target.

On one day in March, $6,000 in cash had been taken from my dad's account. He told investigators he did not want to prosecute. He thought it was only $2,000 and did not want to make a fuss about it.

After the race, my goal was to show my dad the checks made out to the two and get him to understand how much was gone. I wanted to show him the cash withdrawal slips and determine if he had signed them. My dad has consistent in one thing. He has repeatedly said he did not give away all his money. I believed him because my dad is a frugal man, not prone to giving away money. Could I make him understand how much has gone and where it had gone? Could I make him want to pursue an investigation?

We didn't at this point know how we would pay for my dad's care. Giving away all your money usually renders you unfit for government aid. It made me sick to think that two people he thought were his friends had taken advantage of him this way. Would we be able to hold them accountable?

I just wanted to visit my dad and make sure he was OK. Imagine being in a nursing home with no family closer than three hours. Most of his friends have passed away. I know he just wants to go home. When I look at my dad, I wonder if that is how I will be at 81. I am so genetically like my dad. I have his CMT and asthma. Will I get dementia, too? Who will take care of me? Will someone take advantage of me? I am there to protect him and fight for him. Who will fight for me when I am 81?

* * * * *

My mind raced as I waited for the starting gun. As much as I did not want to be there, I needed the distraction of that time between the lines. It is too easy to get defeated and discouraged by the things that happen. Not only did I need the distraction of the race, I had to prove to myself that I could race despite all the distractions.

One of the things being a triathlete has taught me is focus. I put off doing triathlons for years because I was afraid of the open water swim. I remember telling the neurologist who had diagnosed my CMT I thought I would need to change over to triathlons due to my CMT. It was getting more and more difficult to run long distances.

So one day I found myself on the shore of a local lake waiting for my swim wave to start in a local triathlon. I plunged in. I felt like I was drowning, I tried the side stroke and back stroke. I finished, but my swim time was terrible. My next race was not better.

I had a breakthrough when I wore a wet suit for the first time. I no longer felt like I was drowning,, but my problems weren't cured. The first triathlon I did right after Nationals and again had trouble in the swim. I was still reeling mentally from everything that had happened there. I think I was mentally and physically exhausted. I started the swim and the buoys on the course looked so far away. I tried several times to make myself swim the distance. I just could not do it. I was tired, yes, but I am always tired before the start of a race. I was just not focusing mentally during the swim and it was affected my ability to finish.

A short time later, I went to a corporate coaching class. The instructor spoke via video. He had started as a tennis coach and now talked about something he did to improve the tennis skills of one of his students. She was having problems consistently hitting the ball. He told her to say in her mind, "bounce" when the ball hit the court and "racquet" when she hit the ball. Her performance drastically improved.

Immediately, I knew how to change my swim. The mind can only have one conscious thought at a time. So instead of worrying about all the things I normally did during the swim portion of the race, I replaced my worries with my own two-word mantra. "Face … breathe."

To be an effective swimmer you need to have good body position or you do feel like you are drowning. That means putting your face in the water during the swim stroke, so it became "face" and when I turned my head to breathe, I would say in my mind, "breathe."

During the entire swim leg, I repeated my mantra. When other thoughts crept in, I focused and repeated my mantra. It worked wonderfully and I not only swam well that day, but every swim leg since. *Face ... Breathe ... Face ... Breathe ....*

I was focused the entire race. I felt so good about even getting to the starting line and finishing strong. Just like life, I can't control what happens in a race or how well I do compared to other competitors. What I can control is how I prepare, how I focus, and how determined I am to finish. None of that matters if I don't show up and race.

The ability to concentrate and lose myself between the lines has paid dividends. The discipline from the race has carried over to work. I am much more able to concentrate. I found the relief I needed in the distraction of the race. I won't walk away from that so easily again. For me, racing is about staying mentally and physically strong as I battle the effects of CMT.

Chapter 70
In Over My Head

*Move out of your comfort zone. You can only grow if you
are willing to feel awkward and uncomfortable
when you try something new.*
—Brian Tracy, entrepreneur and motivational speaker

The words to *In Over My Head* by The Fray came through loud and clear on my iPod morning of my indoor bike class. After a night in Computrainer class, I felt completely in over my head, too, and it wasn't a good feeling.

To get ready for my next Paratriathlon National Championship, I knew I had to improve my bike leg. The event was held at the end of May 2012. I knew to be competitive I would have to bike during the winter because many of the athletes I compete against live in areas where it is warm enough to bike all winter. Wisconsin winter weather just does not allow outdoor biking.

To get in some bike time, I signed up for a five-month indoor biking class. My bike leg is the weakest part of my triathlon and I decided the off-season was the perfect time to work on it. I know I need to improve because the competition is going to continue to improve at Nationals in Austin. I would be going back to Austin again in 2013 to try to compete in the Paratriathlon National Championship.

The bike class works by putting your road bike in a stand hooked up to a Computrainer. The Computrainer changes the resistance based on the course and workout the instructor plans on the main computer. The workouts are customized based on assessments of the athletes and time trials done throughout the class.

The system readout at the station connected to your bike tells you how fast you are going and your power rating in watts, as well as some other numbers. All sounds good, right? Except your number is posted on a very large screen in the front of the class along with everyone else's numbers. So everyone sees it. I knew exactly how I measured up. As an engineer, I am all about numbers and I don't like it when I don't measure up.

At one session, we did a time trial and I came in last among 12 students. I was at least 2 mph slower and a lot of power less than anyone else in the class.

That was not the worst part. I feel like a complete newbie. Everyone in the class had taken it before. Most of them are Iron Man competitors. They all know each other and what they are doing. I don't even know how to put my bike on the stand or set up the software.

Everyone in the class has been nice and helpful. They helped me get my bike set up. It just seems everyone knows this but me and I am the slowest kid in the class. This discomfort is all in my head, which doesn't make it any less painful.

It is just like school gym class. I feel like I don't belong. Being a competitive runner for years, I know the routine and just what to do. I don't like the feeling of not knowing what I'm doing.

We were doing drills in which we pedaled with only one leg. The coach came along to correct my foot. It was pointing down—because of my foot drop, that is what my feet do. She kept telling me to pull back, but I don't have the flexibility to do that. How I just want to be normal like all the other students in the class.

So all around, I had a bad night. I felt completely out of my league. I thought I would fit in at Nationals, but had been told I was "too strong and not disabled enough." Yet I don't really fit in with other athletes either. I am living in the land between.

My coach tells me not to compare myself to others and she is right. But there is an even bigger issue here. Fear of not keeping up has kept me from joining group rides and runs. Sometimes, I let that fear of being in over my head get the best of me. Not this time.

Despite being in over my head, I went back to bike class the next week and pretty much every week after that. The motto my trainer sends in her email says: "If it doesn't challenge you, it won't change you." That's was why I took the class. I didn't just want to be good enough to win a National Championship in Austin. I want to be the best I can possibly be. I want to show others with CMT what they can do and to never give in to their CMT, even if that means sometimes being in over your head.

Chapter 71

Week 1: Boston II
A Tough Start

Motivation remains the key to the marathon:
the motivation to begin, the motivation to continue;
the motivation never to quit.
—Hal Higdon, author of 34 books on running and runners

This time, the acceptance to the Boston Marathon came almost immediately. I applied on September 15th when registration opened and was accepted the same day. No months of waiting and wondering this time. I was accepted for the 2013 Boston Marathon.

It was a good feeling. Now that I was a Boston veteran, I knew just what to expect. I knew the course and knew what I had to do to get ready.

The only problem, I had an injured ankle.

I had been struggling with injured ankles since just after last year's Boston Marathon and Paratriathlon National Sprint Championship. Hoping they would get better, I had competed all summer. I finally stopped running in mid-September 2012 to get treatment. After being looked at by about a dozen medical professionals, going through an ultrasound and MRI, I was diagnosed with a cyst on the right ankle. The doctor has tried unsuccessfully to drain it. I am getting physical therapy and it has gotten a bit better, but the cyst is still there and still hurts.

It could have been worse. I thought the pain was from tendonitis or a tear, both of which could mean the end of my running career. Either of those would take months to heal, if at all. As it is, I believe the cyst is due to my CMT. The muscles slowly waste away due to slower nerve conduction. The thinning happens in the muscles first at the wrist and ankles. The cyst is from irritation due to overuse. That area is vulnerable because it is where there is muscle atrophy. Lots of those affected with CMT have problems with this area, the peroneal tendon.

The inflexibility of my ankles puts a strain on the outside of the ankles as well. That all adds up to two ankles that are tender and painful. Would I get through an 18-week training program again on two weak ankles?

The problems had started when I switched to clip-less bike pedals for the triathlons for the swim-bike-run events. However, my right ankle was really painful if I bumped the area or it got touched by a massage therapist or doctor.

I asked my therapist about how to deal with it, and he said experiment to see what works. It is rare for a medical professional to see someone with CMT and I have never met one with experience working with an athlete with CMT The lack of available medical advice means most of the time I have to experiment to see what works to treat and prevent injuries. So I started taping my ankles when I biked and ran with hope that the support would add some stability and keep the injury from getting worse.

Every night, I treat both ankles at home with ultrasound and keeping my fingers crossed. To do the treatment, I put gel on the ankle on the cyst on the right side and in the same general area on the left side. The unit is hand held with an electronic switch on the top and a metal disk on the other side. I turn on the unit and run the metal disk side over the injury. The ultrasound waves are transmitted through the gel and the purpose is to speed healing. It does seem to help with the ankle soreness but has not made the cyst disappear.

It wasn't just the injury that worried me; it was what it might mean if it never healed. The cyst is located at the spot at which my lower-leg muscle wasting is most evident. I wondered if the injury was due to the strain of both running long distance and having CMT. I worried that the cyst was a signal I was living on borrowed time as a long-distance runner.

I don't know how much longer my body will allow me to run marathons and half-marathons, or even participate in triathlons. I had already missed several half-marathons earlier in the year as I sorted out this injury. I stopped running for almost two months, which gave me a taste of what life without running was like—and I didn't like it. It was possible the upcoming Boston race might be my last marathon.

Last year, in 2011, quite a bit of publicity surrounded my Boston run. While I will be happy to do any interviews, I won't seek them out this time around. The notice I got did put pressure on me to perform. I felt like I was representing the whole CMT community. Someone at my CMT group told me, "We are all counting on you."

I feel like I proved myself last year and this year I want to enjoy the experience. One thing that won't change is that I will still be raising funds for CMT research.

The Boston fans are the best and I plan on having a good time—if you could call running 26 miles of hills is a good time. I am running this one for me. If I happen to raise a little awareness for CMT and some funds for research, those will be a bonus.

In 2011, I had set a goal of finishing in the top three in my division. I accomplished that. I am going to train hard, but not be too concerned about the results this time. I plan on training hard, but maybe with just a little less intensity and less pressure on myself than last year. I intend to have fun and enjoy my second Boston Marathon experience.

Chapter 72
Week 2: Boston II
Getting Out the Door

Once you learn to quit, it becomes a habit.
—Vince Lombardi

The key to being successful at anything—especially athletics—is consistency. You need to work out on a regular basis. Working out nearly every day can be a challenge. For me, the toughest part is getting started. Once I am working out, I'm fine, so I've come out with a few tricks to get out the door.

Group Outings
The local running club, Badgerland Striders, and the local Triathlon Club offer classes and group workouts. It is much less boring to work out in a group.

I also think the quality of the workout is better. I tend to work just a bit harder when I am running, biking, or swimming with others. With company, the time goes by much more quickly, too.

Partner

When I am in Texas, I run with my favorite running partner, my nephew's dog, Mojo. He gets so excited to get outside, it is contagious. His excitement and the fun we have running together get me motivated to get out the door. Running with a partner or a group can be fun. When training for my first marathon, I met with two friends every Sunday morning at 6 o'clock. There was no time to procrastinate like I do when I run by myself. Having this commitment got me up and running every Sunday morning.

Errands

I started training for Boston 2013 two weeks ago. The long runs are always tough, especially after my two-month hiatus from running. To help me get out the door, I decided to combine the run with doing an errand. I had Christmas cards to mail, so took about time at a time and ran to the post office, which is about 1 1/2 miles round trip from my house. By the time all my cards were mailed, my long run was done. Sometimes I take back library books at the beginning of a run. It is just the little trick I need to get me out the door.

Competition

In the winter, it is cold and it gets dark early. When I get done with work, sometimes the last thing I want to do is workout. Swim workouts are especially tough. I hate getting into a cold pool when it's cold outside. So I think about Nationals in May 2013 and wonder what my competition is doing. I think about them working out to be ready and that motivates me to do a complete workout. I tell myself Beth Price is swimming today (current National Champion). No disrespect to Beth; rather the opposite. I know if I am going to win at Nationals, I can't skip workouts. I know my competition is working out so I had better do so, too.

Classes

I am taking an indoor bike class. The biking section is the weakest part of my triathlon. I signed up for a five-month long class. I never feel like going to class. Still, I go every week because I've paid for it. The money is charged every month, whether I show up or not. This class is tough. Our cadence, watts, and miles per hour are all posted on a big screen in front of the class. Keeping up with everyone else is very motivating.

I also tell myself the tiredness isn't really tired; it is just the CMT—as if that makes a difference. I just feel tired, I'm not really tired. That usually works and actually, I usually feel less fatigue after I work out.

You may find different tricks to get you working out. It does not matter what you do to get you moving as long as you work out.

Chapter 73
Week 3: Boston II
I'm Running as Fast as I Can

No matter how slow you go, you are still lapping everybody on the couch.
—Russell Warren, sports medicine surgeon

Sometimes I don't sleep well, at least not well enough to have dreams. This week on vacation I've been able to sleep in, which means dreams. One strange dream I had was running related.

I'm also watching *Downton Abbey* on my Kindle. *Downton Abbey* is a WWI British drama and I am enjoying it immensely, which may be why it figured in my dream as well.

I dreamed I was doing a speed workout and running as fast as I could go. I looked to my right and saw the character Edith from *Downton Abbey* right beside me. I thought I was running really fast, but she was walking quite slowly beside me. So despite my running as fast as I could, I was really quite slow. Nothing like your sub-conscious to put you in your place.

Usually I don't have a clue what my dreams mean. In this case, I've been concerned about my running speed. The last time I had a long layoff due to injury, my running times went from a 7:15 to 10:00 minutes per mile. So I have been wondering if I've lost even more speed due to the cyst on my ankle.

Every time I think about doing a group run or bike ride, my thoughts include words like, "I'm slow" or "I won't be able to keep up." I usually am not the slowest one, but that fear is still there. In a small enough group, I feel slow and not much of an athlete.

I tried out a GPS watch a couple of weeks ago and my easy pace was 13 minutes for a mile. I had a problem before with this make of watch, so for those two weeks, I have been wondering if the problem was with me or the watch.

I guess I will know for sure when I do a 10-K race at the end of January. It is frustrating and worrisome to watch the effect the progression of my CMT has on my running. I fell twice in the last week, so the reminder of the impairment is always there. I wonder how much longer I can run and if I only run a 13-minute mile, will I even want to.

Recall that I quit racing after my bike accident in 1999 because of the drop in my running times. I was no longer competitive and my feet burned. I came out of retirement when I was diagnosed so I could raise awareness of CMT.

I remind myself I am lucky to even be running and preparing for an event like Boston. I try and remember how far Team CMT has come since its start. Exactly one year ago, I wore the HNF uniform for the first time at a half-marathon in the Dallas area. We have grown to 110 members. On almost any weekend, one of the Team members participates in an event to raise awareness of CMT. I never thought this little team would grow so big and do such great things. All my Team CMT members—you help me to stay inspired and to stay out there running.

Chapter 74
Week 4: Boston II
More Unlikely Heroes

A hero is someone who has given his or her life to something bigger than one's self."
—Joseph Campbell, American author and teacher

One month done in training for Boston Marathon Number Two. I couldn't believe I was actually running after being sidelined for 2 1/2 months with ankle injuries. I did 13 miles for my long run and my coach says she can't believe I can run that distance.

My coach, Joy Von Werder has CMT as well and is an Iron Man Triathlon Finisher. The Iron Man is a 2.4 mile swim, 112-mile bike leg, and a 26.2 mile run. Her CMT makes it almost impossible for her to run now. It amazes me that athletes find the time and have the desire to train for three races that are so long.

I realize how blessed I am to be running at all. What keeps me going is the deep desire to raise awareness and funds for research. I am inspired by what I call our unlikely heroes.

When I started Team CMT, I was told by a national CMT organization that it did not know of any CMT-affected athletes except for me and a triathlete in England. At the time of this writing, Team CMT has 24 CMT-affected athletes. I call them our 24 miracles, since even numerous medical professionals have told me people with CMT can't run.

Patients with CMT were once advised to go home and rest. It was thought an exercise would damage muscles and accelerate the condition. Many neurologists still advise against vigorous exercise, like long-distance running. I have been lucky; all three of the neurologists who have cared for me have told me to keep running if it is working for me.

My current neurologist just had me genetically tested. She is so surprised by my long-distance running she is sure there is something different about my genetics. I could introduce her to three other CMT-affected athletes who have finished Ironman races and several others running long distances. Maybe we have multiple miracles on the team. This week, I had my annual check-up with my neurologist. She knows I run marathons and do triathlons. Not only does she encourage me; she now tells all of her CMT-affected patients to exercise.

Some of my CMT symptoms improved when I started long-distance running. Not all of our athletes are runners. We run, walk, bike and participate in triathlons. Most report an improvement in their symptoms and quality of life.

We are changing the face of CMT. Many of our CMT-affected athletes have inspiring stories. I am so humbled to be a part of their effort. I am so in awe of family and friends who support us and participate in events for us or with us.

Words are not adequate to express how grateful I am for our mission and those who are with us in this fight. We are making a difference!

I am still strong because I have been active my entire life. It's thrilling to know that we are inspiring others to be active. Think about what a difference that is making in the lives of those affected by CMT. Think just by the fact we are exercising, a doctor is going to tell another CMT patient to stay active. Staying active will help slow CMT's progression. We make a difference in the life of every CMT patient taking the advice to stay active.

I belong to several Facebook CMT-related groups and have seen a real change in the conversation in the last two years. Members are talking about the things they do to stay active and enjoy life. We have come so far from the days when doctors told CMT patients to go home and rest.

The other change I see is those affected by CMT are wearing their braces uncovered. Some have talked about how they carry brochures to share when asked about their braces. Maybe they aren't athletes, but they are heroes to me. It takes so much courage to take the risk to be open about our condition. It is so important to get this condition out of the shadows. We have nothing to be ashamed of and nothing to hide. When they choose to be open about their condition, they are heroes. I think the visibility of Team CMT has given them the courage to be open about their condition.

Our other heroes are the families who support us, like 7-year-old Brook O'Connor, who runs for her mom or Lincoln Stultz running for his sister Regan, Megan Seebeck running for his dad, Darell Wright running for his wife and other family members, Kim and Courtney who run for their sister Allison, and countless others. Their support is so important to us. It is so wonderful to see the love they have for your CMT-affected family members.

Then there are the friends who joined the team just because we asked. I think about my friends and countless others asked to join by team members. Their willingness to give themselves to our cause is humbling. Thank you for caring about us. Your efforts to raise awareness are making a difference. Our efforts are beginning to attract the notice of sponsors. We hope to have some announcements soon.

My Computrainer bike class instructor shared with me she saw our Team CMT members at the Racers Against Childhood Cancer Race into the New Year's run at State Fair Park. So don't ever think the efforts go unnoticed. I had shared with her about my CMT because I was struggling to keep up with all the "normal" athletes in the class.

Some team members have joined because they saw our athletes at an event or found us in a web search.

Team CMT members may think they are just running or biking, but you are all heroes to me. It has nothing to do with where your finish or how fast you run. If you have CMT, it is a miracle you are an athlete. If you are a member of our team, you are dedicating yourself to a cause bigger than yourself and that makes you a hero to me.

Chapter 75
Week 5: Boston II Unplugged

*The trail is the thing, not the end of the trail. Travel too fast
and you miss all you are traveling for.*
—Louis L' Amour, American author

'm still running unplugged, meaning I don't run with a
radio or iPod. Because I am not the fastest runner, I have
lots of time to think when I am doing my long run.

This week my long run was 14 miles, which takes me 2
hours and 30 minutes. I guess it's 14 miles because I don't wear
a GPS either. I base my distance estimate on the last half-
marathon I ran in Allen, Texas last year.

Usually long runs for marathon training are done on
Saturday or Sunday. I often try to do them on Friday because it
gives me an extra day to recover.

Sometimes after my long run, I cannot sleep. My whole
body feels like it is on fire and my nerves just feel like the
circuits are overloaded. My legs often twitch and jump like I
am being shocked. So if this happens on a Sunday night, I
won't get a good night's sleep and be ready for work the
next week.

I did not do my long run this week on Friday because I was too tired and it was rainy. I switched to Saturday because there was no rain in the forecast. I had to start early because although it was 51F in the morning, the temperatures were supposed to drop to near freezing by mid-morning. Getting my workouts in depends on weather and making a good recovery.

There was time when I would have just skipped the workout. Many years ago, I was a member of the Milwaukee Rowing Club. I was rowing that summer with a rower from the University of Wisconsin. We were preparing for a national competition in St. Paul. One afternoon, Ann and I decided it was too windy to go out on the Milwaukee River. As we were leaving, we bumped into one of the club's many experienced rowers.

When we told her we weren't rowing, she said something I have always remembered: "What if it's windy on race day?" She was right. You have to work out under all conditions. You never know what the weather will be like on race day. The Boston Marathon last year was proof of that. Good thing with the temperatures soaring to 90 degrees, I had had plenty of experience running in hot temperatures.

So whenever I can, I run outside in all kinds of conditions. I really lucked out today. It was 51F when I got to my running spot at 8 a.m. Weather in Wisconsin can be almost anything, but 51F days in January are a bit rare. I picked out another new course and was ready to have some fun.

Milwaukee is on Lake Michigan, one of five of the Great Lakes and the only one entirely inside the United States. The lakes contain 20 percent of the world's freshwater supply. I am lucky enough to live in Milwaukee with extensive running paths along the lake.

Today I parked at Discovery World where the *Dennis Sullivan*, a replica tall ship, is moored in summer. Milwaukee was once one of the busiest ports in the U.S. The schooner was built to educate about Milwaukee's maritime history.

It was sunny, but oh so windy as I ran north. Winds were about 40 mph. I have great views of the water. It might be hard to believe but the water of Lake Michigan looks different almost every day. Some days it smokes, others it is gray and stormy. Today it was sapphire blue.

The USAT age group National Championship in 2013 and 2014 will be in Milwaukee and the run portion will be held in the same area as my run.

I did some speed work and a few loops around the Milwaukee Art Museum. The museum was designed by world-famous architect Santiago Calatrava. The museum is meant to resemble a ship under sail, another nod to our maritime past. I was done with my run before I knew it.

Another fun run and it has really worked to change up my running routes. I enjoyed the scenery and the wonderful sunny day. Running is supposed to be fun and running in a different place has made my workouts really enjoyable again. On a long easy run, I can enjoy the scenery, do a little reflection and enjoy the experience. All important for getting out the door the next time. Plus when I run into wind, heat, snow, or almost anything else on race day, I will be ready because I've done it in workouts. All important for feeling confident no matter what happens on race day. If it's windy in Boston, I'll be ready.

The weather forecast for the evening was for 1-3 inches of snow. Running in the snow is fun as well, but tomorrow is a pool run/swimming day.

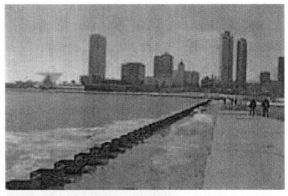

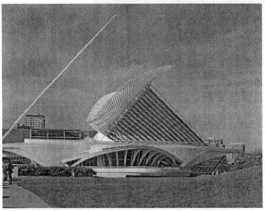

Running along Lake Michigan with the Calatrava Art Museum and the Milwaukee skyline

Chapter 76

Week 6: Boston II
A Change of Scenery

Perseverance is just as important as talent.
—Joan Rivers

G etting ready for a marathon means lots of running. The long, easy run is one of the keys to preparing for a marathon because it teaches your body to run long distances.

I had a 13-mile run on my schedule this week. Because I'm not a fast runner, it takes me almost 2 1/2 hours to cover that distance. I woke up Saturday and it was 20F. My inner debate began. It was cold, I was tired, and I was fighting with myself doing the workout.

Could I take the day off? No, I had taken the day before off. Could I switch my long run to Sunday when it was supposed to be warmer? No again. I had a tempo run scheduled for Monday and I don't like to run two days in a row.

I mentally went through my running route starting from home. Honestly, after twenty years of living in my neighborhood, I was bored with my usual routes.

Because it was cold, I thought about doing a treadmill workout. The office in which I used to work out was now closed, which meant going to another location at my company's downtown office to train. It is a hassle to park downtown and get through security in the building.

After winning the argument about working out at all, I thought I would go to downtown Milwaukee and do at least an hour outside, and if it was too cold, hit the treadmill in our downtown office.

I parked near my company's downtown headquarters. I planned to run for 60 minutes, head back to the car and grab lunch in the form of an energy bar, and then decide if it was treadmill time.

A few blocks into my run, I saw the entrance to the Riverwalk the city has built along the Milwaukee River. It stretches for three miles along each side of the river. Perfect! It was just what I needed—even in the dead of winter, the picture I held in my mind was one of summer. Hundreds of people sit on the outdoor patios at the bars and restaurants. In winter, the area is deserted. The river was beautiful with lots of ice floes, and there were lots of shops and restaurants to look at.

As I ran, the temperature climbed to 33F and there was no wind. Downtown Milwaukee is a bit of a ghost town on the weekends. There was virtually no traffic as I crossed the streets. I went up and down both sides of the river.

Part of the run took me into the old Trostel Tannery site. The tannery was one of three in the city at a time when Milwaukee was the largest tanner of hides in the country. Anyone who grew up in Milwaukee remembers the distinctive smell of leather and worse the tanneries emitted until they closed in the early 90s. The area now has trendy bars and condos. I also got into the Brewer's Hill neighborhood, which is built on hills and overlooks the river and downtown. It was a neighborhood I'd never seen. The new scenery made the time go really fast. It was an hour and 15 minutes before I returned to my car. I finished the workout with some speed work and a trip through the Third Ward area of Milwaukee, another old warehouse district converted to condos and shops. Before I knew it, the 13 miles were done. I had so much fun. I was on a runner's high the entire day. It is amazing what a change of scenery does. I am going to run downtown again and seek out some new areas. I hope this week's run is just as much fun and goes just as quickly.

Chapter 77

Week 7: Boston II
Polar Chick

It is not the strongest of the species that survives or the most intelligent; it is the one most adaptable to change.
—Charles Darwin

Throughout this book, I've talked about being consistent in workouts to be successful as an athlete. Well, this week I had to be consistent and adaptable.

My coach Joy Von Werder sent me the tee shirt with a picture of a runner that said "Polar Chicks." She had them made up for the athletes she trains in Florida. Florida cold is no way near as bad as Wisconsin cold. She tells me it's freezing when it's 40F down there. The Florida folks think they have it tough. We are pretty hard core up here in Wisconsin. We start breaking out the shorts and sun screen at 40F. For us, that's a January thaw.

Joy is a great coach—she really lifted my spirits with the gift (shown opposite).

On Monday night, when it was time to do my 8-mile tempo run, it was 6F and icy. It was definitely time to hit the treadmill.

My problems were not over. My workout clothes had been sitting in a frigid car all day, so I had to figure out what would be the least uncomfortable to put on first. I started with the socks, then the shorts...all like ice. I was hoping the jog bra would have warmed up a little. No such luck and the orthotics in my shoes were like blocks of ice. However, like me, the cold clothes warmed up quickly and I got my workout done on the treadmill.

It was still 6F when I hit the pool for a swim workout a few days later. Think about trying to get into a pool when you are cold and it's way below freezing outside. The pool building where I swim is lined with a wall of windows. When it is cold outside, the pool water gets really cold. I get in the hot tub first

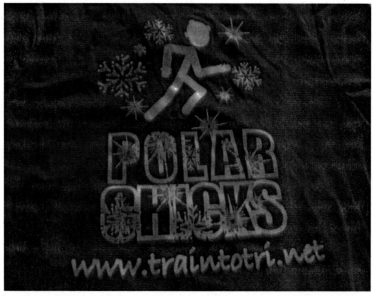

The Polar Chicks T-shirt from coach Joy Von Werder for chilly days in Florida..

to talk myself into getting into the cold water. Sometimes the hot tub is the only place I feel warm all day.

Because of my CMT, I always seem to be cold. My hands and feet always seem to be cold. When I get into the pool, the water feels like ice and it takes me at least four laps before I start to warm up. The hot tub before and after gets me through the laps.

I had to do my long run of 16 miles on Friday because I wanted to run a 10K race on Sunday and choose not to do hard workouts back to back. It was still 6F outside, which meant another treadmill workout, so I gritted my teeth and put in 3 hours and 5 minutes. There was no TV in the workout room. So, yes, it was just a boring as you might imagine. I did some speed work and looked out the windows and soon I was done.

The treadmill only goes for an hour so I had a little break between each set. Doing three sets sounds lots better than three hours. Thinking about this workout as three short runs with some speed work was just the mental adaptation I needed to get through.

I felt sick on Sunday and was still very tired from the long run, so I had to do some more adjusting. I skipped the race and just did a very easy run near home. This week was all about adapting both to the cold and the tough workouts.

The really tough part of my training is coming now. The long runs will soon be 20 miles. My body will adapt if I give it lots of rest and change my workouts as needed.

I'll get to Boston with consistent workouts and just a little bit of adaptation.

Week 8: Boston II
A Little Perspective

I found my heart upon a mountain I did not know I could climb, and I wonder how many other pieces of myself are secreted away in places I judge I cannot go.
—Laurel Bleadon Maffei

There's a saying in Wisconsin if you don't like the weather, just wait a bit. We can see just about any type of weather at any time. Last week was no exception. Here is what we had for weather last week:

Monday—43 F and sunny
Tuesday—58 F and rainy, flooded streets
Wednesday—12 F and all that rain turned to ice
Thursday—6 F and -20 F wind chill
Friday— - 2 F and -25, -30 F wind chill
Saturday—13 F and windy
Sunday—a balmy 18 F and sunny

I am entering into my highest mileage weeks. My long run was 17 miles this weekend (3 hours and 20 minutes) on the treadmill because of the ice and cold. It always takes my body some time to adjust to this work load. My normal CMT tired rose to marathon workout tired.

Although I get one day away from working out, I still get extremely tired. Training kicks it up a notch.

The tough workouts make me a strong athlete once my body adjusts. Kind of like all the cold weather makes Wisconsin people tough.

Being down physically also drains me mentally. I know it isn't normal to go to bed exhausted at 7 p.m. A little perspective helps. I have been through this before and know my body will adapt. It will all be worth it when I cross that finish line in Boston.

I also know I'm lucky to be running and preparing for an event like Boston. I remember the 22-inch snow storm we had Feb 2nd just three years ago. The weather can be lots worse than we saw this week.

March is just three weeks away. Soon it will be warm enough to run outside all week long. Both Boston and spring will be here before I know it. This winter and touch training shall pass.

2013 started with a new job, my first job change in almost ten years. Soon I will be starting a position as Manager for Business and Process Improvement, with my new company's power plants to develop procedures and improve their operations.

After ten years in my previous position, I will have to learn a new business, faces, and names. I was comfortable, knew the routine, and had a great boss. Any new job carries risks. But if I let a little risk scare me, who knows what opportunities and experiences I might miss. Unless I test myself, I will never know what I am capable of doing.

As an athlete, I've learned the value of pushing myself and taking risks. Sometimes I've tried things, not knowing if I would be successful. When I crossed the finish line of my first marathon, I felt like there was no limit to what I could do.

Sometimes others put limits on what they think we can do. Sometimes the biggest limits we have are the ones we put on ourselves. There are many in the medical and CMT community who think we can't or shouldn't exercise. I won't let anyone place that limit on me.

Being successful at work or as an athlete is the result of a few simple things: attitude, activity, and focus. Attitude has to do with what you believe about yourself and what you tell yourself is possible. When I believed I could run the Boston Marathon, I focused on that as my goal until I found a way to get in.

The focus and activities then shifted to preparing and successfully completing the event. I am glad I did not let fears and doubts hold me back. What an experience I would have missed if I had.

We have many athletes on Team CMT who have completed marathons and Ironman triathlon events. Like me, they have discovered that when you have a passion for what you do, whether it is your job or a mission, the results can be amazing.

So, yes, I am a little nervous about the new job, but I won't let that hold me back from learning everything I can and doing my best.

Chapter 78

Week 9: Boston II Winter Wonderland

Instead of giving myself reasons why I can't,
I give myself reasons why I can.
—Wally Amos, American entrepreneur, author, founder of the
"Famous Amos" chocolate chip cookie brand

The long, easy run is the bread and butter of a marathon training program. It teaches your body to run for long mileage and in my case, being on my feet for a long time. It really helps if I can get outside to do my long run. Treadmill work is tedious.

This week, my long run was only 12 miles, which took me about 2 hours and 10 minutes. We had a fresh layer of snow on Friday morning and I was all set to do my long run after work Friday night. It was 32F and there was just a slight breeze. That afternoon, the weather was perfect for a run.

When I first started running in the winter, I was surprised how comfortable I stayed. Running on Friday meant the longest workout was done and I could relax for the rest of the weekend. Workouts were still on the docket, but they would be easier.

Running in the winter can be really beautiful, especially right after it snows. The trees and everything else were coated with 8 inches of fresh snow. It was the same storm system that dumped over 30 inches on Boston and 40 inches in other parts of the East Coast.

There is a park right across the street from my house. Every neighborhood in Milwaukee has a neighborhood park. It was all part of the plan by the city founders to make it a great place to live.

This is the kid's playground. I am sure the sledding hill was busy, but the playground was deserted. I run in the park often and like to see all the families enjoying the playground. So I had some beautiful scenery to look at. The pictures do not do it justice. There is nothing more fun for me then running on new snow. Most of the sidewalks had not been shoveled yet. Running on 8 inches of snow is like running on a sandy beach. It does not feel like work at all.

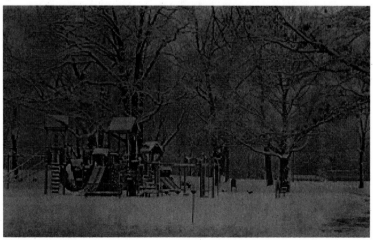

The Winter Wonderland across the street from my house.

City of Milwaukee workers are really efficient about removing snow. A storm of 8 inches is easy for them. Between plowing and salting, the streets are down to wet pavement in 24 hours. Their efficiency creates a challenge of its own: big piles of plowed snow lie at each corner and it's not always easy to climb over them.

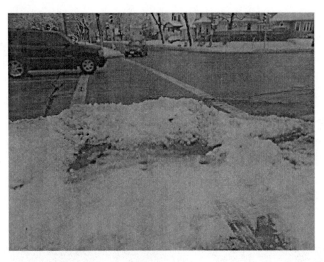

I used my run to mail my fundraising letters so I had a purpose. The post office is about a two-mile round trip from my house, so six trips back and forth made those 12 miles go by pretty quickly.

Runs like this help me to remember why I am a long-distance runner. They give me the "why" to get out the door the next time I have to do a run.

Come March, snow and winter get pretty old, but those first few snows are really beautiful and fun.

Chapter 80
Week 10: Boston II
Long Goodbyes

Vitality shows in not only the ability to persist,
but the ability to start over.
—F. Scott Fitzgerald

The 18 weeks of training for a marathon don't happen in a vacuum. Lots can happen in those 18 weeks that can help or hinder training. At the very least, I have to work my training program around the other events in my life. These last few weeks have included two milestones and two long good-byes.

Leaving my previous job has meant a long month of goodbyes for my three client work groups, as well as three going-away parties. I also spent the last month training my replacement and tying up work projects. Part of that process was saying goodbye to a work area in which I'd spent the last ten years.

The second good-bye came earlier in the month. I've been a member of the National Ski Patrol at Crystal Ridge for 23 years. Crystal Ridge became the Rock Ski Area earlier this year. I expected it to be a learning experience for the new hill management. We had new patrol leadership as well, and decisions were being made that I felt put both injured skiers and patrollers at risk. I expressed my concerns and did not see any effort to resolve the issues.

When I found myself the only Ski Patrol member on a Saturday night shift with no safe way to transport an injured skier, I knew it was time for a change. I am in the process of looking for a new patrol home. It was a tough decision to leave behind so many great people. I let both hill and patrol management know the reasons for my leaving. Hopefully my departure will be a catalyst to improve safety, especially of the patrol operations. You never know; I just might be back. So it has been a season of change and adaptability, two key skills for an athlete.

Change can be good, exciting, and difficult all at the same time. It brings new challenges and you have to let go as well. Change comes as part of the marathon training program as the mileage builds and workouts get more challenging. I am just getting to the point in my training program where the workouts are almost more than I can handle. Change in our lives prepares us for what is ahead. Change is not always easy, but it is necessary. I believe the things that happen to us in life prepare us for the next bend in the road, just like workouts prepare an athlete for a race or game day.

My workouts this week included an 8-mile tempo run, a long run of 19 miles, a race, and a bike time trial.

Everything went well until Saturday night, when I woke up at 12:30 a.m. I was wide awake and unable to get back to sleep. I immediately knew there was no way I was going to do a race and my long run on the same day. I had planned on making the 6-mile race part of my 19-mile run.

I cancelled any thought of doing the race so I could sleep in a couple of more hours. When I got up at 8 o'clock that morning, the temperature was 9F. It was supposed to get up to 28F. My run was going to take four hours. If I waited until it warmed up, would I get my run in before dark? Off to the treadmill I went.

I made a bargain with myself. I would do half inside and half outside. I got started and while I was in the gym, I went ahead and did the entire workout on the treadmill. Four hours on a treadmill with no TV, just the radio. Yes, it is as boring as it sounds. By my reckoning, I ran about 19 miles. At least I am hoping it is.

That workout completed my training for the week. One more week closer to Boston. One week closer to spring and hopefully warmer temperatures. I'm not sure I can handle many more weeks of 4-hour treadmill workouts.

The key to change, whether in a workout plan or in life, is to stay flexible, work the plan, and to be confident you will be ready and prepared for the next bend in the road

Chapter 81

Week 11: Boston II
Runner's High

It is not the disability that defines you; it's how you deal with the challenges the disability presents you. We have an obligation to the abilities we do have, not the disability.
—Jim Abbott, Major League baseball pitcher born with one arm

Before I became a runner, I scoffed at people who talked about the "runners high." I thought, How come if running is so much fun, you never see a runner smiling?

Well, there is such a thing as runner's high. After a tempo run or speed workout, I feel great for hours. I get euphoric on some of my long runs, especially in the fall with the colors or on newly fallen snow in early winter.

Well, I've not had a runner's high the last two weeks. I am in the toughest part of my training program now. There are just 7 weeks to go to Boston. On Saturday, I did a 9-mile tempo run, followed on Sunday by a long run of 20 miles. That is just the way running is. Sometimes it's fun; other times it's just hard work.

So I am a little down physically and mentally. After a weekend like this, I still have to get up and go to work.

Still, relief is here.....this training week is an easy week. On the agenda are a 6-mile tempo run. That seemed easy and fun even as tired as I was. I got a tiny bit of a runner high. I surprised myself by doing this run on almost no sleep.

So why do I do it? Why do I work so hard? I do it because there are people with CMT who would give their right arm to run even one mile. I am in pain for a few days; there are people with CMT living with life-altering pain every day. I work this hard because very soon, there may come a time when I can't. I cherish every mile I am able to run. I run for those with CMT who can't. So pain or not, sleepless night and all, I am going to keep running.

I work this hard because when I run that course in Boston and see the crowds, it will all be worth it. When I cross that finish line, all the pain and sleepless nights will be forgotten.

Just like I know all the money I raise and the awareness the members of Team CMT raise will help to find a cure and I know it will all be worth it.

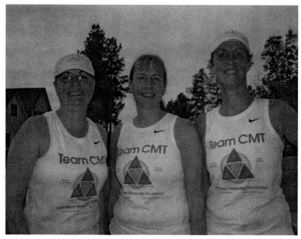

Team CMT members Barb, Courtney, and Kim

Chapter 82

Week 12: Boston II
Finishing Strong

*Victories in life come through our ability to work around
and over the obstacles that cross our path. We grow stronger
as we climb our own mountain.*
—Marvin Ashton, publisher and business man

WEEK 12: MARCH 3, 2013

This week was an easy week . Easy being a relative term since now even the easy weeks include lots of running and cross training.

It's so important to finish every work out and every week well. A good ending to the week sets me up for the next week of training. Finishing is strong whether in training or in a race. I had an awesome finish to my week of training. On Friday night, I did 13 miles on the treadmill (2 hours and 20 minutes). It felt good and the treadmill miles per hour setting has gone up quite a bit.

Even better, on Saturday, I attended the Dare2Tri workshop in Highland Park, Illinois. I almost didn't go. I thought people would look at me and wonder why I was even there. Despite having CMT, I know I look fairly normal. I cleared my attendance with the organizer. Some organizations that work with paratriathletes do not work with athletes in my paratriathon (TRI 3).

Dare2Tri was founded to help train triathletes with physical challenges. TRI 3 paratriathles have neuromuscular conditions like MS, cerebral palsy or like me, CMT. I wanted to be sure it was ok for me to attend when I might not look like I have an impairment.

The day did not start off well. The directions I got off MapQuest were all wrong. I called the event organizer and she got someone to talk me in.

Right away, I met my volunteer assistant for the day. Marissa is a nurse at Northwestern Hospital. She works with patients with neuromuscular conditions and actually knew all about CMT. She was really interested in how it affected me as an athlete. She is herself a triathlete and has qualified for the USAT Age Group National Championship in Milwaukee. It

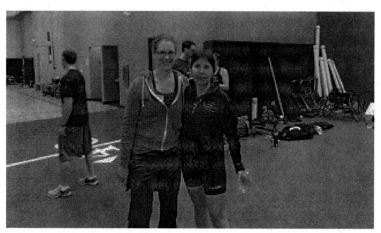

Marissa, my volunteer assistant at the Dare2Tri workshop.

will be her first real trip to Milwaukee and I know she is going to love the course. I look forward to cheering her on.

As my assistant, Marissa was there to help me with anything I needed for the day. She got my bike all set up in the bike stand for the Computrainer class. She was also my photographer all day. Thanks, Marissa. It was great meeting you.

The day started with yoga (love it) and next up was a swim clinic. It was the best single hour of coaching ever. I came away with lots of new drills. The coach pointed out that I was not bending my elbow. When I said, "I know and how do I fix it?" the coach had a drill. Great to have things to practice in the pool.

The pool so warm it felt like bath water—a nice change from my club pool where it takes four laps to even start to warm up. Lots of laps and the hour-long swim clinic was over before I knew it.

Then it was on to running drills. We learned all kinds of drills for warming up and improving our stride. Finally we finished with a Computrainer class. I had missed my Milwaukee class on Wednesday, so this was a great catch-up. My legs were dead from my treadmill run, so I just dialed things back a bit. I don't look one with the bike, but it was a good workout.

I even got to ride next to Melissa Stockwell, the current Tri 2 National Triathlon Champion. That was the very best part of the day.

Melissa was the USAT paratriathlete of the year in 2010 and 2011. She is a multiple Tri2 National Champion and is also a level 1 USAT Triathlon Coach and co-founder of Dare2Tri based in Chicago.

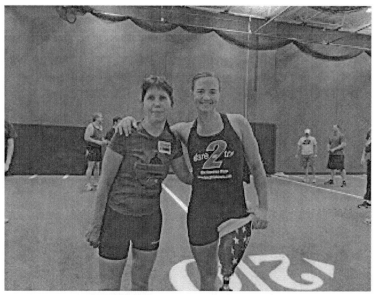

The author with Melissa Stockwell, co-founder of the Chicago Dare2Tri and current Tri 2 National Triathlon Champion.

Melissa could not have been nicer and we talked a bit about last year's nationals and my experience there. I am looking forward to meeting all the athletes again at the Paratriathlon National Championship in Austin. It was really a thrill to meet her and be in the same group.

It was good to be practicing in a group of athletes with challenges. Everyone was great to me and I can't wait to see them again in Austin in May. I am really glad I went. It was a fantastic experience, I learned lots and finished the week strong.

Sometimes I am not sure where I belong as an athlete. I can't keep up with "normal" athletes and get tired of being the slow, clumsy one. Before going to the workshop, I didn't know if I would fit in with a group of challenged athletes. Everyone was so friendly and accepting. Thanks, Dare2Tri, for making me part of your family. Thanks for letting me finish out my week by meeting lots of amazing athletes. You inspire me!

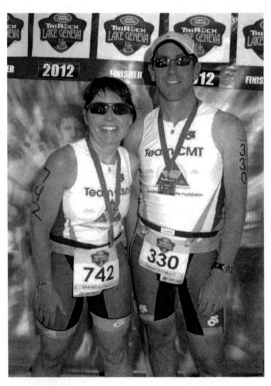

Team CMT at the TriRock in Lake Geneva, WI

Chapter 83
Am I an Athlete?

Every successful person in life began by pursuing a passion, usually against all odds.
—Robert Kiyosaki, investor, author of *Rich Dad, Poor Dad*

On one of my visits to my family in Dallas, we were headed out to dinner to celebrate my nephew's college graduation. I was sitting in the back of the car talking with my two nephews, Brandon and Dan. I said something about being an athlete. My nephew Dan started laughing. Not a little chuckle, but doubled over with laughter at the thought of me being an athlete.

I guess the image of me as an athlete was just so funny to him; I am just their middle-aged, weird aunt. So I asked what makes someone an athlete. Do I have to be like Tiger Woods or Aaron Rogers to be an athlete? I admit I may not be the picture of athletic grace, but I do have had some athletic success.

I told my nephew I was the National Champion in the Open Division of the race I had been to in Austin. He was suitably impressed. So I gained a little bit of street cred with that accomplishment. He was not impressed by my 2nd place finish in my division in Boston.

So what is an athlete? Merriam Webster dictionary defines an athlete as: *A person who is trained or skilled in exercise sports or games requiring physical strength, agility or stamina.*

Well, I may not be skilled, but I am certainly trained as a runner and triathlete. If time and expense mean anything, I am an athlete. I train six days a week, sometimes in multiple sports if I am getting ready for a triathlon.

Most of us with CMT struggle with being defined as athletes. We still carry memories of awkward and clumsy moments in gym class. But I think if you have a body and you use it to run, swim, bike, and walk, then you are an athlete. We know what it means to suddenly turn an ankle or trip without a moment's notice. We lack the fine motor control and grace that marks the average athlete.

If expense is any measure, then I am a world-class athlete. For instance, here is what it cost me to get ready for the Paratriathlon National Championship in Austin in 2013:

Road bike: $3400 (needed new one to be competitive)
Bike fit and accessories: $660 (shoes, computer, pedals, parts)
Massage: $720 ($60 per month)
Chiropractic treatment : $1200 ($200 a month for 6 months)
Coaching: $1920 ($160 per month)
Bike class indoor: $575 (5-month class + 1 month hill class,
  Compu-trainer)
Qualifying race: $100 entry fee
USAT Membership: $45 (required to compete)
Bike tune-up: $95
Tri Club Membership: $45 (free classes and clinics)
Nationals entry fee: $65
Plane to Austin: $484

Genetic Test $300 (prove CMT to assessors)
Hotel Austin: $352
Meals Austin: $60
Gas to Austin: $50
Case to transport bike: $359
Bike pack/re-assemble: $100
Bag fee for bike: $70
Running shoes: $130 (one pair, go through 4 or 5 a year)
Swim goggles: $69
New uniform: $92 (custom Team CMT uniform)
Gym membership: $36 per year
Swim Clinic: $40
Wetsuit: $130
Transition mat: $30
New helmet $95
Total $12, 032

Triathlon is an expensive sport, especially when competing at the national level. My expenses won't be that much every year. I bought a new bike in order to be competitive. My first year at Nationals, I rented a bike and beat the time of the national champion by about ten seconds. I was later assessed a time penalty for losing my number, which gave me a time 30 seconds longer than hers.

Some of the equipment, like a wetsuit, goggles, and transition mat are not a yearly expense, but must be replaced occasionally. Triathlon events on average cost $100 for each event. USAT events, which I need to qualify for National competition, are more expensive.

I knew if I wanted to compete on that level, I would need to ride a better bike. That is a one-time expense. Some expenses are consistent, like the massage and chiropractic/physical therapy treatments. Because of my CMT, I have really tight muscles in my legs and this leads to injuries. So treatment is a constant part of my life as an athlete.

Going to a national event like Austin means travel and hotels. I had to buy a bag to transport my bike. To qualify for the next national level event, I must travel to a regional competition in Omaha. So that means more hotel and travel expense. At least Omaha is within driving distance from Milwaukee and I won't have to take my bike apart or pay for it on the plane.

So if training and expense make an athlete, I think I qualify. I did not spare any time or cut any corners in getting ready for my second experience at the Paratriathlon National Championship. I was will to do it to feel well prepared and do my best. I was representing Team CMT and the CMT community. I knew winning a national championship would be great to raise awareness of CMT. Training and equipment were just some of the preparations I made to get ready for the competition in Austin. I also had to prepare for my classification appointment with the assessors.

First, it's on to Boston …

Chapter 84

Week 13—Boston II
Expect the Unexpected

Nothing feels quite as exhilarating as meeting a challenge.
—Dr. Yosiya Niyo

TRAINING WEEK 13: MARCH 10, 2013

This week and next are the two toughest weeks in my marathon training program. Workouts include a long run of 20 miles and a tempo run of 13 miles.

Tempo runs are always tough for me because they are meant to be run at my current 10K race pace, and it takes me almost two hours of hard effort to finish this workout.

Long runs can also be a challenge, but since they are run at a pace about two minutes per mile slower than a 10K pace, they are much more relaxing than a tempo run.

We had another snow storm this week and the sidewalks are icy. Same challenges, new week. It is a challenge to get in training around snow storms, work schedules, and my CMT.

Saturday, I had the challenge of getting in a 20-mile run. That means running for 3 hours and 50 minutes. The weather report said 40F and maybe some rain. As I went out the door, I could see the telltale drops on the driveway. I shuddered at the thought of a long run on the treadmill, so outside it was going to be.

I thought I'd better get some practice running in rain, just in case it rained on race day. So it was off to the post office to mail a few bills and then to my brother's house to drop off a letter.

After running for about 90 minutes, I came home to change my wet clothes. While at home, I got the dreaded knock on the door from my tenant.

"Could you look at something," Sandy asked. me.

"Sure," I said, because it's in the landlord's job description to keep the tenant as happy as possible.

"Well," she said, "I think there is a bat in the house," and pointed to our uninvited guest hanging from the backdoor curtain. It was hard to even tell what it was at first. Bats are not good to have in the house since it's possible they carry rabies.

After a little thought, I came up with a plan and enlisted Sandy. I put down a quilt and gave her a rug. I knocked down our visitor with a broom right onto the quilt, and Sandy threw the rug on top. I scooped up our uninvited guest and took it outside. Done, no man needed. I may sound brave, but if it had been a snake, I would have packed, sold the house, and moved.

Once I changed, I headed back out the door for the rest of my run. I needed something to distract me so I decided to run past the first place I lived in my neighborhood.

Milwaukee is divided by neighborhoods. I live in Bay View, which once had the largest steel rolling mill in the world. It was a mill town until it was annexed by the City of Milwaukee in 1894. Since my house was only two blocks from Lake Michigan, I also decided to head off to take a picture of a place I used to work. To get there, I cut through the grounds of St. Francis Seminary.

St. Francis Seminary was built in 1855. The tree-lined driveway is really beautiful in the fall. The school educates priests and lay workers for the Catholic church. Church offices are right next door. Cardinal Timothy Dolan would have had an office there when he was Archbishop of Milwaukee. Cardinal Dolan later became the Cardinal of New York and was mentioned as a candidate for pope. The view from the top of this building is stunning. I was up there on a tour one fall.

My next stop took me to my previous workplace. The building lies on a cliff rising above the shores of Lake Michigan. My cubicle was on the top floor on the Lake Michigan side, so I got to see the changing moods and colors of the water every day. The inside was a palace with Oriental rugs, antiques, and hardwood floors in every conference room, and had cost millions to build. It might be one of the reasons the company went bankrupt. I was one of many losing who lost their jobs when that happened.

I love running the bike path along the lake. My final stop before I turned left away from the lake was the South Shore Pavilion. I had not carried water with me Saturday, so the Pavilion was great for a water stop and bathroom break. South Shore Park Pavilion was built in 1933 with Depression-era relief labor paid for by Federal program called the Civilian Conservation Corp. You can still see projects built by the CCC all over Wisconsin.

A few more laps around my neighborhood and I was done. So despite rain, icy sidewalks, and a bat, I was able to finish my run. I felt a huge sense of accomplishment to have another 20-mile run on the books. Just one more next week and I will start tapering my training regimen. If I adjust to the unexpected during my training runs, I will be ready for anything on race day.

Chapter 85

Week 14—Boston II
Dress Rehearsal

There is not time to think about how much I hurt;
there is only time to run.
—Ben Logsden, runner and author

This is the toughest week of my Boston Marathon training program. For the 2nd week in a row, I had a long run of over 20 miles.

Every week, the Boston Athletic Association has been posting training tips on Facebook. This week, it suggested that the last long run be a dress rehearsal for the race. Nothing should be new if possible on race day. Every long run is really practice for race day. You practice using the fluids and food you will use on race day. An athlete will try to mimic course conditions in his or her long run.

While you can't predict the weather, it's also a good idea to wear the same clothes during the long run you plan to wear on race day. It's better to find and solve any problems in practice. Poor socks could cause blisters, clothes may be make you too hot or not keep you warm enough. Seams could chafe and cause problems. You want to find any problems in a shorter rehearsal race. If you make a mistake in your clothing or shoes on race day, it can be a long and painful day.

Things that are minor irritants like a shirt with a seam that bothers you are no big deal in a 5K because you are done in less than 30 minutes But running a marathon takes me over five hours. So that little seam rubbing would be with me all that time. Such a "small" thing might make the difference between finishing or having to drop out of the race.

Running a dress rehearsal also helps to give peace of mind also means knowing you have accounted for every possible problem ahead of the race. You do not want any surprises on race day. As an athlete you test out what you will eat and when as well as what you will wear.

On Saturday, I lined up for the Luck of the Irish 10K in Hartland, Wisconsin. The race started close to my Boston race start time, around 10:30 a.m.. The 10K was just part of my long run for the day.

The race also gave me a chance to do a practice run for race day with Robert Kearney, who would be one of my guides in Boston. As a Mobility Impaired runner, I am allowed to take two guides to assist on the course. Robert would run the first half of the course with me and Cheryl Monnat would take the second 13 miles into the finish.

Robert and I had a nice run and chat together during the Luck of the Irish race. I knew the slow pace would keep me out of the medals and it did, though I finished one place out of the medals.

Teammate Cheryl Monnat finished 2nd in her age group and 2nd over all for her age group for the series. Cheryl did not run with us because she was in contention for the overall age group award for the series.

I took a short break after the race and then headed out the door again to finish my 20 miles. When I run longer than 2 1/2 hours, my legs hurt. Saturday both ankles were also hurting. So I wonder if it is so painful to run 20 miles, how I will ever run 26 miles on race day. Somehow, I always do. I call it "Race Day Magic." I'm going to need that magic at least one more time when I run Boston II.

Hooray! The toughest part of my training is behind me. I can now begin decreasing my mileage every week until race day. I am looking forward to having some extra time as my workouts get shorter.

Chapter 86
Running Diva

Be yourself. An original is always worth more than a copy.
—Unknown

I t was no secret I would be running the Boston Marathon again. I'd been blogging about my training for months and posting status updates on Facebook. Boston will be marathon number eight for me. Unlike most of my marathons, I will have company.

At Boston last year, I joked that Cheryl and Robert were my entourage. They had traveled to Boston to share the marathon experience with me. This year, I would put them to work as my guides. I could use the help and I thought my friends would enjoy the Boston experience. They have tried twice but have not made qualifying times yet.

Their job will be to carry my water, gels, and anything else I need. Long-distance runners expend so much energy, they need to eat when they run or risk "hitting the wall" or running out of energy. Most runners use sport products that come in gels, bars, jelly beans, or blocks. They are easy to digest and get the energy into your system quickly. I use gels, blocks, and beans. The beans are just like jelly beans, the blocks are like Gummy Bears and the gels are like a pudding. I eat two to three gels every hour or suck on the beans.

Since my wave starts at around 10:30, I would be running through lunch, so I also needed a protein bar to eat at lunch time. That is a lot of stuff to have along. My guides will carry all of it and hand me fuel or water when I need it. Other jobs include photographing the experience and talking to me to keep me from getting bored.

I told my sister this and she said I sounded like a diva. So I had to look up the meaning of diva. I found two:

This one from Webster's dictionary: *An unusually glamorous and successful female performer or personality. A true diva will do anything to get anything she wants.*

This one from the Urban dictionary: *A bitchy woman that must have her way exactly or no way at all. Selfish, spoiled and overly dramatic.*

My sister was joking and I hope I don't fit either of those definitions. I will have to check with my guides. I think of a diva as someone who loves attention and the limelight. That is not me at all. I prefer to be in the background.

I am single-minded and determined. I did not let anything stop me until I realized my dream of running the Boston Marathon. So now I am doing it for the second time and hoping to raise another $10,000 for CMT research.

I appreciate Robert and Cheryl's help. I am falling more frequently now when I run, so they will be there in case I get hurt. They will also provide much appreciated moral support. In addition, they were the first two members of Team CMT. I am so excited to have them share in the Boston experience.

Running half the marathon in Boston will help them prepare for a half-triathlon for both of them in July and a full Iron Man for Robert in November.

So, am I a running diva? Well, maybe just a little bit. But don't tell anyone.

Chapter 87

Week 15—Boston II
Stranger in a Strange Land

Don't wish it were easier, wish you were better. Don't wish for
fewer problems, wish for more skills. Don't wish for fewer
challenges, wish for more wisdom.
—Earl Shoaff, entrepreneur known as the "Millionaire Maker"

I started a new job about a month ago. I'd been in the same department for ten years, and now moved to a different division of my company. It is like working for a brand-new organization. Sometimes I feel like I'm in a foreign country. I don't know anyone, don't know my way around, and I feel like I don't know the culture. I was in a meeting last week and everyone arrived 15 minutes late. They were all old friends and laughed and talked, leaving me completely out of the conversation. That has happened more than once in the last month.

This is not the first time I've experienced such behavior at my company. When I started the job I just left, I reported for my first day. The guard did not want to let me in because, well, I was a stranger. The administrative assistant came and led me to my cubicle. My office area had half walls so I could see the entire operating area. There were three large operating areas with about six people in each area. Not one person talked to me or even said hello all day.

My new co-worker had the cubicle right next to me. At about 1 p.m., he said to me, "Did anyone show you around or show you where the ladies room was?" I said no.

He said, "Oh," and went right back to his business.

I took it upon myself to introduce myself. Good thing I am pretty independent. I figured things out on my own and ended up being very successful. I expect to have the same experience in this assignment. It will just take some time to figure things out.

My journey as an athlete sometimes has had the same feeling. I never expected to be running an event like Boston even once, much less twice. It seems a little strange to be traveling to Austin for the second year to compete in National Championship for the Paratriathlon. I was the open division champ last year. Champion and my name have never been said in the same sentence before. Sometimes it feels like Boston and Austin are happening to someone else, a bit surreal.

I never expected when I started Team CMT that it would grow so big or have so many CMT-affected athletes. All of this has been unexpected, but is certainly not unwelcome.

So my journey as an athlete will continue. Training for Boston has gone smoothly. I had my last long run of 13 miles. Now I start the taper. The taper feels strange as well. After weeks of long mileage and intense workouts, I'm cutting the mileage back to nothing before the race. It feels strange to have so much extra time as the workouts decrease. Before I know it, I will be standing on that start line in Boston.

Now that is a feeling I am familiar with.

Chapter 88

Week 16—Boston II Excitement

*A good laugh and a long sleep
are the two best cures for anything.*
—Irish Proverb

The Boston Marathon really starts to seem real when the runner's packet arrives in the mail, announcing the 117th race. It is exciting to get it. Just two weeks from Monday, I will be lining up on the starting line for the second time.

This year there is a runner's passport. It has a map of the city, sites, tickets for pre-race and post-race parties. Most importantly, it contains the card I need to pick up my race number.

The packet included the clothing catalog. One of the perks of running Boston is being able to wear the Boston Marathon jacket after the race. I never wear the jacket before the race; that's considered bad luck. Completing the race and wearing the jacket is a great way to let everyone know about your accomplishment.

I have last year's jacket. I am not crazy about the orange and black color scheme. Orange is my least favorite color.

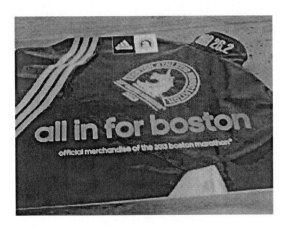

I plan on wearing that jacket on the plane and all over Boston before the race. It marks me as a Boston veteran. Considering how brutal the course conditions were last year, I wear that jacket with considerable pride. I am very proud of the finish and my 2nd place in the Mobility Impaired Division.

The 2013 jacket is blue and yellow. A big improvement over the orange and black from last year. I plan on buying lots of Boston Marathon clothing.

The last piece of information was the runner's booklet. It has everything a runner needs to know about race weekend. This is my second time at Boston, so it's all routine now. Still a nice souvenir to have.

It was a good week. I am on a taper now. My workouts have been cut by over half. I really like the extra time and energy I have. I filled the time with appointments to my chiropractor and massage therapist.

This is the healthiest I have been going into a marathon, with just the injury to my right ankle. Hoping the taper will help that heal a bit.

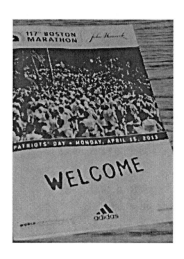 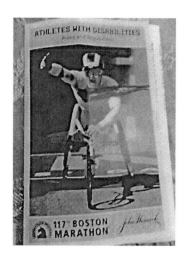

I had some extra time and energy to socialize this week as well. I started the week with the Tri Wisconsin kick-off party. Tri Wisconsin is the local triathlon club in Milwaukee. It was fun to meet other athletes and talk about upcoming races.

Wednesday night I closed out my five-month indoor bike class with a wine and cheese party. It was fun to socialize with the classmates I have been riding with for months. I even got to talk to some of the cute guys I have had my eyes on.

My long run this week is 8 miles, which seems really easy compared to the 20-mile runs I have been doing.

Throughout the entire training program, I have also been swimming and biking to get ready for the Paratriathlon National Sprint Championship on May 27th. It will be no time before both races are in the books.

Chapter 89
Week 17—Boston II
Flying Under the Radar

*To finish will leave you feeling like a champion
and positively change your life.*
—Hal Higdon

T he race is less than a week away. I always pack the
weekend before I leave. That gives me time to get any
needed items and adjust what I am taking. Often during
the week, I think about something I forgot to pack and add it to
my luggage. If I wait too long to pack, I know I would forget
something important. Besides, after work, making dinner and
getting in a workout, I usually do not have much energy left for
anything else. I have a list of everything I need to take to be
sure I don't forget anything. Weekends are when I get most
things done.

Once I am packed, I can start to get excited about the trip
because I am ready. Last year, I was really nervous, because I
felt I carried lots of expectations, both the ones I put on myself
and the ones from the CMT community.

When I pack for Boston, the first thing I do is get all the
race gear together, two pairs of shoes and socks (because I
change at the half-way point), running skirt, Team CMT singlet
(if it is warm), long running pants, and a long sleeved shirt to

wear under my singlet in case it's cold. Spring weather in New England is unpredictable, so you have to be ready for anything.

I also pack all my gels, water bottle, sports drink, and energy bars I will use along the course. For protection from the sun, my sun screen, hat, and sun glasses. Finally the vanity items to look good for pictures, make-up and a nice colorful headband if it's cloudy and I don't need a hat.

The first year I ran Boston, there was a Team CMT fundraiser so I brought along a number of Team CMT items to give away to the crowd, things like water bottles, beer glasses, mouse pads, notebooks, and so on.

The rest of the packing is pretty easy, I pack the things I would take for a casual weekend—jeans, some shirts from other marathons, some nice sweaters, and of course my Boston Marathon jacket.

Wearing the jacket is pretty cool, especially if you've run the race before. It is fun to go to the airport wearing your Boston Marathon jacket and see other runners wearing theirs. It means you are a member of a very exclusive club. My running friends and I never wear a shirt from a run until we've crossed the finish line. The same holds for the Boston jacket. Bad luck to wear it before you cross the finish line, but worn with a real sense of pride once you are a Boston finisher.

Last year, there was a lot of media attention pointed my way, so I felt I had to run really well. I set a goal of placing in the top 3 in my division, and accomplished that with a 2nd place finish in the Mobility Impaired Division.

The experience was even better than I imagined. I still remember running the last mile and feeling the volunteer put the finisher medal around my neck. I had worked so very hard for that moment. All the hard work and sacrifice were worth it.

It will be a different Boston experience this year. I chose to keep it low key. I didn't seek media attention, although I would have done media if offered. I wanted to enjoy this Boston race, with no pressure and no expectations. I wanted this Boston to be fun, well, as fun as a marathon can be.

I know the course now and won't be intimidated by it. My qualifying marathon in Madison, Wisconsin in May 2011 was tougher than the Boston course.

Also, I did not train as hard this year. I over-trained last year and ended up with a cyst on my ankle. I still have it and am hoping to get through the race. I am also focused on the Paratriathlon Nationals in Austin at the end of May. Because of that I have done more swimming and less running. I hope I did the right amount of training.

Boston will be fun this year because two friends are accompanying me as guides—Cheryl and Robert. They will split the course and each run a half-marathon. The company will be very appreciated. There will be times during the race when I will so tired and in so much pain I will want to quit. Their presence will help me be strong. I know Monday will be a tough day. Marathons always are. I am so thankful for their support.

I hope everyone with a wish to run Boston sees that dream come true. Qualifying for and running Boston really has been a life-changing experience. I once thought my dream of running Boston was out of reach. I know determination and hard work can take me as far beyond anything I might hope for and dare to dream about.

So yes, this Boston will be low key, but no less thrilling and satisfying

Chapter 90
Pre-Race Boston II

*I thought about how many preconceived prejudices would
crumble when I trotted right along for 26 miles.*
—Bobbi Gibb, the first woman to finish the Boston Marathon 1966

Bobbi Gibb was denied entry into the Boston Marathon in
1966 because she was told women were not capable of
running more than 1 1/2 miles. Amateur rules at the
time forbid women from running anything longer than that in
competition.

She ran in 1966 anyway, sneaking into the race. She
electrified the running world by finishing in 3 hours and 27
minutes. She beat 290 men in the field of 417.

Bobbi Gibb changed the perception of women and racing.
Efforts like hers paved the way for changes for woman in sports
and in larger society. She showed the world what women could
do to make changes happen for other woman. She was one of
many pioneers who paved the way for women of my generation. I am sure even she did not realize the effect of a simple act
of running a marathon.

Those of us with CMT doing runs, walks, rides, and
triathlons, are pioneers as well. People with CMT were once
told to go home and not exercise. I still hear from members of
the CMT community that working out too hard is bad. They

were once told hard exercise would accelerate their disease. When one of our CMT affected athletes asked the CMTA to start a running team she was told "No, people with CMT can't run." Many in the CMT community put limits on themselves and what they think they can do.

Now they have a team of their own and tell their members to be active. Event by event, we are changing notions about what CMT-affected athletes can do. As I read posts on Facebook, I see many people with CMT now talking about exercising. Exercise is so important for staying strong and living a full life with CMT. We have already made a difference! Team CMT members should be proud of the part they've played.

Members of this team have done events that are a challenge for any athlete. Three of our team members have done Ironman Triathlons, many run marathons and half marathons. We are showing the world what someone with CMT can do. When I found out I had CMT, I could not believe that 155,000 other Americans had this disease. That is as many as have MS. I could not believe I have never heard or CMT. I could not believe so many others were not aware of this disease. That did not seem right to me. I set to change that with my efforts and those of my Team CMT teammates.

Tomorrow in Boston, there will be 500,000 spectators. That is half a million people who will see the Team CMT singlets on our three members running this event. Raising awareness puts a face to this disease. Raising awareness is the first step to raising funds. In a marathon the finish line seems far away.

Sometimes it seems like treatments and a cure are far away as well. I know with hard work we will get there. I know the members of Team CMT are a large part of that battle. Running a race like Boston may seem like a little thing, but I know some how it is all connected to our fight for treatments and a cure. Just like the finish line, it can't come soon enough.

When I was getting a chiropractic treatment a few weeks ago, the doctor remarked "I had a whole team working on me." I laughed and said "It takes a whole team to keep me going." I also have a whole team behind me.

Thank you to the members of Team CMT. We are in this together. You inspire me. I will be thinking about you all as I run tomorrow. Thanks also to coach Joy Von Werder—you answer my endless questions and you keep me calm and centered.

I wonder if Bobbi Gibb had doubts when she ran Boston or if she had any idea of the effects of her run. Sometimes the simplest acts can have the most profound influence. I know I have doubts every time I line up for one of these events.

Chapter 91
Boston II—Race Dedication

A man of many companions may be ruined,
but there is a friend who sticks closer than a brother.
—Proverbs 18:24

I always dedicate my marathon runs to someone. It helps to motivate me and get me through the miles. When I dedicate the race to someone, I feel like I can't quit or I am letting them down.

My first marathon I ran for my nephew Brandon. The Madison Marathon was my first Boston qualifier and I dedicated it to my mom, who had recently passed away. The Marine Corps Marathon I used to qualify for Boston II, I dedicated to all the members of Team CMT. Last year, I dedicated my Boston run to HNF President Allison Moore and Team CMT member Joyce Kelly.

This year, I am dedicating my Boston run to my friends and guides, Cheryl Monnat and Robert Kearney. They say when bad things happen in your life, you find out what you are made of. That may be true, but I've found you also find out what those around you are made of.

I have friends from high school who I have not heard from since the day I announced I had CMT. I have siblings who have never acknowledged my CMT. Cheryl has been there for me from the very beginning of my quest to qualify for Boston. She was there when I first talked about forming Team CMT. She listened patiently as I talked about my CMT. She looked at endless designs for our Team CMT singlet. She has run in countless races, usually far ahead of me. If I asked her, she would run right beside me.

Cheryl has provided much-needed support throughout my racing and training. In Madison, she was there in the last mile to cheer me on when I needed it most. Last year in Boston, she was at mile 16 and mile 25. I don't think I could have finished without her support. She truly has been a friend who has been closer than a sister. We have known each other since we pledged to the same college sorority, Alpha Omicron Pi at UWM. She has shown the true spirit of sisterhood when I needed her most and I am forever grateful. Cheryl has the rare ability to be excited and thrilled by the success of others. She has never been jealous of the media attention my efforts have earned.

Cheryl and her fiancé Robert Kearney were the first two members of Team CMT. They ran our debut race in Brown Deer, Wisconsin, in April, 2011. Robert and Cheryl have continued to faithfully run races and ride in bike events for the team, even when I couldn't due to injury last year.

Robert agreed to be on the team and has run in events just because I asked him. That says a great deal about the type of person he is. I remember one of the first times I met Robert, Cheryl and I were running in a half-marathon and he was doing the 5K at the same event. He said Cheryl and I were hard core. He has run countless events for the team, including the Dublin

Marathon as part of a recent trip to Ireland. Robert is hard core now, too.

He will be my other guide on Monday. I am grateful for his friendship and support, especially since he makes my friend Cheryl so happy.

My friends stick closer than a brother and a sister. I am so proud we will all be representing Team CMT in Boston on Monday.

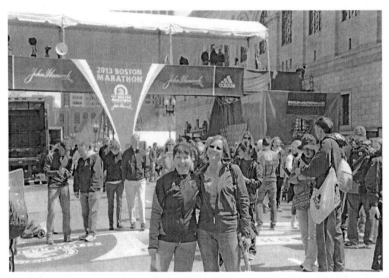

The author and Cheryl Monnat at the finish line before the 2013 Boston Marathon

Chapter 92
Boston II—Post-Race
Witness to History

*Every experience no matter how bad it seems, holds within it a
blessing of some kind, the goal is to find it.*
—Buddha

Tragedy on the Boston course. Two explosions rocked
the finish line. It could not have happened in a worse
place. The area is lined with bleachers. I talked to a
runner who had been a 10th of a mile from the finish. She saw a
trash can explode.

Reports of three dead. My hotel is right next to Mass
General hospital, where they are taking victims. Sirens are
everywhere.

Cheryl and I heard about the explosion when we were at
mile 23. Cheryl had her cell phone and it kept going off with
text messages. We were getting news updates as well. She was
getting texts from friends and from Robert, who had run the
first half of the course with me.

We kept running, not knowing if the reports were true.
More messages asking if we were okay.

Cheryl and I encountered a road block and race officials
at mile 25.5. We were told the race was over and were directed

to Commonwealth Avenue. Nothing more. Thanks to Cheryl's cell phone, we were aware there had been an explosion with reports of deaths and injuries. We were not sure how true they were or the exact location of the explosions. We kept running, hoping the problem was minor and the finish line was still open. It was not. Sirens and emergency vehicles were everywhere.

It was mass confusion trying to find the buses with our luggage. Several times on the way to find our luggage bus and when standing in line, we had to move aside for emergency responders coming down the street. A sea of people moved down Commonwealth Avenue. It was all very intense, but quiet and orderly. Most had no idea of what had happened.

At the bus waiting for our luggage, we talked to a woman who had been a tenth of a mile from the finish when the first bomb when off. She did not finish. We heard later that one of our friends had been in the first aid tent when the bombs went off. He was a veteran runner, but made the mistake of not drinking enough water; he was seeking medical attention in the same tent into which the dead and injured were brought.

I parted ways with Cheryl after I collected my luggage, since she and Robert were staying at another hotel near the Boston Commons. She told me later she had a hard time getting there because the area had been blocked off as a crime scene.

My lodgings were at the John Jeffries House, near Massachusetts General Hospital. As I walked back to my room, I watched the people around me. Everyone was somber and quiet. The main questions being asked were, "Where were you?" and "Did you finish?"

As I walked, I came to a group all dressed in white marathon jackets with blue piping. I knew the athlete's jacket was blue with yellow piping and the volunteers wore jackets that were reversed. I was wondering who these official-looking people were when I saw the ID lanyards hanging around their necks identifying them as medical staff.

All looked grave and all were silent. I asked them if they were okay. They said everyone they knew was all right, but that some of their colleagues had been in the first aid tent when the victims started coming in. They said it was pretty gruesome. I left them as I entered my hotel. My guess is they were headed to the hospital to help out.

The day had been going well and I was running strong. The crowd support was so incredible. This is one of the friendliest cities I have ever visited. My heart bleeds for this city and this tragic event.

I changed guides at mile 13. Guide Cheryl Monnat could only get to mile 16 and had to run back to 13. We had to wait over ten minutes and then some time to change over. Her fiancé Robert was a bit upset. I kept saying, "It's okay." This day was about having fun. Those 10 to15 minutes kept us farther away from the explosion. We heard about it at mile 24. I would have been fairly close in another 15 minutes.

Robert was on the subway on his way to the finish line when the bombs exploded. He had to walk seven miles to get back to his hotel.

When I got back to my hotel, I looked at my cell phone for the first time. I had messages from one of my co-workers and my coach. I texted my co-worker and called my coach.

Then I spent the next 90 minutes emailing everyone I could think of and posting on Facebook that I was okay. A frantic e-mail from Concord resident and college friend Viktor asked if I was okay and to please call him. I emailed back that cell service was out, but I was okay. He asked if there was anything he could do. I told him no, I was okay and safe at my hotel.

I had stayed in Cambridge the year before. Today, the bridges to Cambridge were closed for a time, preventing those staying there from getting back to their hotels. Hotels along the finish line were locked down because it was a crime scene. Dozens of runners were locked out of hotel rooms and many Boston residents opened up their homes to the stranded athletes. The people of Boston have the best hearts in the world and it is why I love the city so much.

The local Milwaukee running club, the Badgerland Striders, was taking roll to be sure everyone was okay. 400 runners from Wisconsin participated in Boston. I posted I was okay and a few minutes later, got a Facebook message from a reporter at Milwaukee radio station WUWM asking if I would do an interview. I briefly talked to the reporter. All this before I had a chance to shower or get anything to eat.

Police were asking people to stay home. The hockey game tonight was cancelled.

Wearing my new 2013 Boston Marathon jacket, I went to a pizza place down the street to grab a slice. When I saw anyone else wearing a jacket, the conversation was always the same: "Did you finish?" and " Where were you?" I just needed to talk about it. I think others felt the same way. I had stopped in the hotel lobby before going out and had similar conversations with runners there.

I went home and watched the TV coverage for hours, unable to break away.

What will I remember from that day? Not that I did not finish.

I will remember all the little kids so eager to give me high fives. I don't know who was more excited about the race. I will remember the students of Boston College on the Golden Mile. So many high fives. I will remember the women of Wellesley. They love to play with the crowd. When I told them they rocked, they cheered louder and provided a needed boost.

All along the course, there were so many little kids handing out cups of water and oranges. I will remember a little boy not more than 5 who held a single gummy bear in his hand. As I passed, he turned to his dad and said, "She took my gummy bear." I almost cried it was so sweet and innocent. I did not really want or need a gummy bear, but he was so cute I just had to take it. I put it in my mouth and told him how good it was. He treated me like I was an elite runner. Well, so did everyone in the crowd.

I will remember the generous spirit of the people of Boston both before and during the run. They are the ones who make this such a wonderful event. I am so sad it was marred in this way. But I think the people of Boston will bounce back strong. I can't want to see it for myself.

After I got back to Milwaukee, I put together a few thoughts about my 2013 Boston Marathon experience.

Chapter 93
Processing Boston

Let not young souls be smothered out before they do quaint deeds and fully flaunt their pride.
—Vachel Lindsay, American poet

When I did an interview last year with a local Boston radio station, I told the audience Boston was my favorite city (outside of Milwaukee) and I meant it.

I had visited Boston for the first time when I was just out of college, bringing with me my freshly minted chemical engineering degree and hoping to land a job with one of the local consulting firms. I had two interviews, but the economy in the early 1980s was worse than today. With double-digit inflation and unemployment, companies were laying off employees, not hiring.

I spent my time between interviews exploring Boston. I stayed outside the city so I even got to experience Boston driving. I walked the Freedom Trail, took in a ball game at Fenway Park, and wandered around the neighborhoods of Beacon Hill and the Back Bay. I fell in love with Boston and since my first visit, it has been a special place for me.

My second visit was just a few years later to attend a professional conference. The professional society running the conference held a 5K race along the Charles River. I took 3rd in my age group, my first running medal ever. That visit, I stayed in the Back Bay area in a lovely bed & breakfast owned by a retired school teacher.

I returned again last year to run the Boston Marathon, the accomplishment of a long-held dream. I vowed that this year's Boston would be a celebration. I would have a good time and put no pressure on myself. I wanted to really remember the experience because with my CMT, I never know if a race I run will be my last.

After Cheryl, Robert, and I picked up our numbers at the exposition area, we went to check out the finish line, since it was just a few blocks away. We took pictures, being careful not to step on the line. We all agreed it was bad luck to touch it until you cross on race day. Runners are a superstitious group. We don't wear race shirts or our Boston jackets until we have finished the race.

As I looked at the finish line the Saturday before race day on Monday, I couldn't shake the bad feeling I had about this race. I always write a blog entry the day before a race and I always end with "See you at the finish line." I left that out this year because the feeling was so strong that I would not see the finish. When one of my friends asked me if I was excited about the race, I said, "I just wish it was over already." I could not shake the feeling that something was going to go wrong.

I wondered where the negative feelings were coming from, because I was healthy and well trained. This was my 2nd Boston and I knew what to expect.

Usually I carry gels, sport beans, and a sports drink with me. I had forgotten my bag of goodies at the hotel. When I realized I had forgotten my race supplies, I relaxed because I thought that had been the glitch for the day, and took advantage of food offered by race spectators.

Since Marathon Monday is Patriots Day (a state holiday), the course is lined with families. It is a long tradition in the small towns along the course to come out and cheer the runners and offer support in the form or water, ice, oranges, and candy. The course is lined with homes and whole families come out to cheer. It is not unusual to see a picnic or grill going in the background. It is a celebration in anticipation of the warmer weather after a long New England winter. It reminds me of some of our festivals here in Milwaukee. We know all about long winters here in Wisconsin.

Another glitch happened when Cheryl, my second guide, was not at the halfway point for the change. The trains did not reach mile 13 and she had to run the additional three miles to meet us, causing about a 20-minute delay. I was not even worried because this Boston race was about having fun and here was a really big issue. I thought this has to be it and now I can finish the race in peace.

We were on mile 23 when Cheryl started getting text messages about what was happening. She got so many concerned texts from friends and family that we stopped so she could answer them.

We were diverted off the course and learned that the race had been stopped. We were about 25.5 miles into the race. We continued to run, not realizing the extent of events at the finish line. We ended up running 26.3 miles by the time we stopped.

In a blink of an eye, the 117th Boston Marathon was over.

This race experience was such a contrast what had happened along the course throughout the race. I remember all the kids lined up on the route. So many little kids all along the course, holding an orange in their hand or a cup of water to give to runners. When I gave them a high five or took what they offered, their faces would just light up.

Lots of runners dashed off the course for a quick hug from friends and family. There were family and friends supporting runners all along the course. My friend Cheryl met me at 16 miles last year and surprised me by popping up after the 25-mile mark, just before the turn onto Boylston Street. Many family members try to be at the finish to see their runners cross the line. One of my guides, Robert, was going to try to get close to the finish line to see us come in.

I interacted so much with the crowds I felt bonded to them. Last year, they had loved me as a runner and this year I loved them back. It made my 2nd Boston experience even better than the first.

I was hit so hard by what happened. Martin Richard, an 8-year-old local boy, was killed as he waited for his dad to cross the finish line. He was just like the thousands of kids I saw lined up along the course. His mom and sister were with him and both were critically injured. It could have happened to any of the kids I saw along the course.

The bombing was such an evil act, contrasting with all the good I had witnessed that day. My heart goes out to the families who lost loved ones and to everyone injured on Monday. Such a senseless act that will change lives forever.

My friends and I had never been in danger. If Cheryl had not been delayed, we would have been on pace to arrive about five minutes after the first explosion. It is impossible not to be affected by those who lost their lives or were hurt. Those bombs could have gone off at any time. Life is fragile. Things happen that you never planned.

If the bombs had been planted at the start of the race, there would have been even more death and injury. Runners were packed shoulder to shoulder between metal barricades. I shudder to think about the panic that could have happened if a bomb had gone off there. I would stand no chance in a stampede.

There was no happy ending for me or many of the other runners. It is estimated up to 16,000 runners were still on the course when the race was stopped. No finish line victory, no finisher medal, no finish line celebration for me or those runners. No sense of accomplishment for a goal met.

When I saw runners at the airport wearing their finisher medals, I felt angry. I felt they were rubbing it in that they had finished and were celebrating a day when such tragic events occurred. It seemed out of place. I understand they may have been wearing their medal out of support. It wasn't rational to be angry, but I was.

When I got home to Milwaukee, I did an interview with a local television station about my Boston experience. The reporter asked me if I would go back and run Boston again. I would go in a heartbeat. I would love to be there in 2014 to show my support.

I am still trying to sort out the myriad emotions about my experience at Boston this year. I hope they catch those responsible soon. No punishment can possibly repair the damage done to the families affected by this incident. Words aren't adequate to describe the emotions I feel.

I hope to go back and do what runners do next year. When you meet another long-distance runner, an instant bond forms. We understand the strength and discipline it takes to train for and complete a marathon. It is what we do.

Writing and running are how I handle stressful things. I hope that running in Boston next year to support all of the communities along the route. What I can't put into words, I hope I can demonstrate by returning and running the event again. Runners are strong and we can be strong for the people of Boston. We can show them we understand and feel their pain. Although we cannot erase the events of Monday, April 16, 2013, we can do what runners do—overcome obstacles, sometimes against all odds.

We are strong and will be strong for the people of Boston. They really are the greatest fans in running and deserved so much better than what happened on Monday.

I also did a radio interview for Milwaukee Public Radio. The next day, a TV crew for a Milwaukee station met me at the airport as I returned from Boston. I am surprised how many people heard the radio and saw the TV interview.

It's a bit ironic I got more media exposure by accident than when I had a publicist the year before. Not the fault of the publicist; it is usually really difficult to get media attention and I got it without intending to. I am sorry about the circumstances that led to the attention.

Someone once told me that people either grieve all at once or a little bit at a time. I fall into the "little bit at a time" category. As I was finishing this book, I got my monthly copy of *Runner's World*. The issue was dedicated to the Boston Marathon. A picture of the finisher medal with a piece of black tape over it was on the cover. The medal is the same one mailed to me a few weeks after the event.

As I read stories of runners and the many tragic injuries, I got tears in my eyes. I feel the same way every time I read through what I've written about the experience. I was never in any danger. No one I know was hurt. I think about how painful it must be for those who were affected. The Boston Athletic Association has announced those of us who did not finish will be invited back to complete the race. I will be back and I will be there to support the people of Boston because I do feel the pain and hurt inflicted on that day.

Chapter 94
Getting Ready for Nationals

Arriving at one goal is the starting point for another.
—John Dewey, American psychologist and educational reformer

I competed at the Paratriathlon National Sprint Championship for the first time in 2012. It was a bit of a fluke I was even there. My Team CMT teammate Joyce Kelly had signed me up for a triathlon in Denton, Texas, in July of 2011 when I was making my yearly summer visit to my family in Dallas. At the time, I had not done a triathlon in over a year and on a rented bike I got a qualifying time.

I was under-prepared in more ways than one. I had done fewer than six triathlons and had spent the months before the race preparing for the Boston Marathon. I had just six weeks to get ready for Nationals after preparing for Boston.

When I went to my classification appointment the first time, I had not known what to expect. I was not prepared when they asked me how my condition affects me in the three triathlon disciplines of swimming, running and biking. I was surprised by the question. I thought, Why are they asking me? Don't they know? They're the medical professionals?

I stumbled through an answer and I don't think I did a very good job of presenting my challenges as a CMT-affected athlete.

So in 2013, I vowed I would be better prepared. I put together a letter of all the ways CMT affects my athletic performance. In addition, I enlisted the help of Dr. Robert Chetlin, an exercise physiologist at the Medical School at the University of West Virginia. He does research on the effect of exercise on CMT.

Dr. Chetlin put together a paper on the effects of CMT on athletic performance and how to assess a CMT-affected athlete. He cited papers that served as the basis for the International Triathlon Union assessment guidelines.

Dr. Chetlin and I compiled research papers on how to assess athletes with CMT. These documents showed nerve conduction tests should be used to assess impairment. I needed to show 15 percent in one arm or leg. The reduced nerve conduction causes muscles to weaken and tighten. My muscles are so tight in my calves my ankles do not have normal flexibility. My ankle flexibility is -8 degrees in my left. This reduced function means I cannot apply the strength I do have in my legs. My physical therapist told me you lose 5 to 10 percent of athletic ability for every degree loss of flexibility.

I also brought with me copies of my genetic test and my nerve conduction velocity tests. Nerve conduction velocity tests are used to diagnose CMT and assess damage. The test measures how long it takes for a nerve signal to travel down an arm or leg. My test showed more than 15 percent impairment.

The manager of the USAT Paratriathlon had several conversations with Dr. Chetlin. She promised to pass all our information on to the assessor. She also promised I would be assessed based on the evidence we would present.

I touched based with Dr. Chetlin the day before I left for Austin and asked him what he thought my chances were. He said if the promises made were kept, I should pass the classification exam.

So I was hopeful as I headed to Austin. I stayed at the host hotel where the assessments were done in one of the ballrooms. I got an email to come down about 30 minutes early for my 6 p.m. assessment. I went early because I had dinner plans with my brother and sister-in-law, who had come along to watch me compete.

I brought along copies of my tests, research papers, and a confirmation letter from the Muscular Dystrophy Association, stating that CMT was one of the conditions under their umbrella.

The assessor really did not want to see them and was a bit dismissive when I mentioned the documents. I was asked questions about my age, how long I had been doing triathlons, and how many triathlons I have done in the last year. I am not sure why any of that mattered since I met all the requirements for being in Austin.

The TRI3 assessment went almost exactly the same way as the year before. I had just gone through an identical assessment by a physical therapist in Milwaukee about a week before Austin when I went to a local sports medicine clinic to get treatment for the same ankle cyst I had been fighting for a year.

The difference was the therapist here in Milwaukee actually used some strength when he assessed me. The assessor in Austin used no strength; a baby would have pushed harder. It made me think she had her mind made up before I ever walked in and planted the thought that the entire process is a complete sham. Those with MS get in, but those with CMT do not. Once more, I was not taken seriously and was dismissed and discounted.

The TRI3 assessor said I was clearly impaired, but she could not qualify me under International Triathlon Union standards. I later found out she was not ITU-certified. I was told to be patient and wait until next year because the standards were being revised. I had been told the same thing the year before.

The fact I presented genetic tests and medical tests showing more than 15 percent impairment did not matter. It did not matter I do not have enough flexibility in my ankles to walk correctly, much less swim, ride a bike, or run.

As I left the assessment, the manager of the event said to me all perky, "You are still a triathlete! You still get to compete in the Open Division." I was angry. I reminded her of the promise made to Dr. Chetlin—that I would be assessed based on the evidence I would present. The evidence included genetic tests proving I had CMT and nerve conduction velocity tests and EMG tests showing impairment.

I shared my feelings on the assessment. I do not understand how athletes with MS with very similar performance times get in, but I do not. How can I be too strong, when the Canadian and World Champion at the event in Austin can do a 22-minute 5K? My time is very close and even better than the National Champion. MS is very similar to CMT. I felt it was the assessor's ignorance about CMT that was keeping me out. I belonged in the competition and was being excluded for no good reason.

Chapter 95
Racing Angry

*Champions are not made in a gym. Champions are made from
something they have deep inside them, a desire, a dream, a
vision. They have the skill and the will. But the will must be
stronger than the skill.*
—Muhammad Ali, world-class boxer, Olympic gold medalist and World
Heavy weight boxing champion

I had come to Austin to race and I was going to race. I was
disappointed and angry to have been shut out of the
National Championship Triathlon for the second year in a
row. I would have no chance for the U.S. team or the World
Championship in London.

I felt like I had been led to water and not allowed to drink.
All year, I had been posting times in races that were better than
those of the national champion. I think I would have walked
away from the whole event if my brother and sister-in-law had
not been there. I did not want to waste their time by leaving, as
much as I was tempted to.

Instead, I decided I would race just as hard as I could to
show the USAT my abilities. As required, I racked my bike in
the transition area. I remember asking a guy I met there if he
was looking for the pro section. It turned out he was a
paratriathlete and I think he was a TRI 3 as well.

I asked him about the assessment process and before I could get the words out of my mouth, he said the process was a farce. He had been classified in and out several times.

My family went off to the Congress Street Bridge. The bridge is famous in Austin for the bats that come out at sunset.

I did everything else I always do the night before the race. Back at the hotel, I laid out my race clothes, put on my race number tattoos, and made sure everything was packed in my race day bag.

The race tattoos are kind of cool. I always see the pros wearing them in race pictures. They are your race numbers and you apply them by dipping the paper the numbers are on in water and then rubbing them on your body. Every race is different. For most races you have your race numbers on your upper arms and at least one calf. Your age or wave number is then written on the back of one of your calves. Once the tri tattoos were on, the only thing between me and the race was a good night's sleep. I was in bed by 8 pm.

I took an Ambien because I can never sleep the night before a race without it. I woke up at 3 a.m. to hear my brother snoring. He had woken me up the night before and this night, it was so loud I could not get back to sleep. I was desperate for sleep so I took another Ambien.

That was a big mistake. My sister-in- law woke me up at 5:30 a.m. I got up to leave and she asked me if I was okay. As I walked to the transition area to set up, I knew why. I was stumbling all over the place. When I put on my wet suit for the swim portion, I began throwing up.

A volunteer asked if I was okay and told me I had my wetsuit on inside out. He helped me get that straightened out. I had overdosed on Ambien. Now I know why they tell you not to take one unless you can sleep for six hours.

I made my way to the swim start. I remember asking how the sprint course was marked. I swear I started with my wave when the race started.

I checked my watch when I got out of the water and it had not recorded my time. I started the watch. The bike and run course flew by.

Because I was no longer in the National Championship Division, I decided to take my Boston Strong duck on the run portion of the race. The ducks are a fund-raising and awareness raising effort for the Boston Strong fund. The ducks have been sent all over the country and are being posted on Facebook.

Since I was not in the national championship wave, I took my little duck along because he fits in the palm of my hand. I have course pictures of me during the run carrying my duck. Posting the pictures after the race would also help raise awareness since I was wearing my Team CMT uniform.

When I finished the race, my watch said 1 hour 23 minutes. I figured about 11 minutes for the swim would put me at around 1 hour 34 minutes.

When I looked at my official time, it said 22 minutes for the swim and 46 for the bike. The race organizers said I did not leave with my wave but left 7 minutes 39 seconds late. In my Ambien-induced state, that is possible. My net time was 1 hr 39 and some change. I remember leaving with the horn for my wave, but who knows.

I had finished second in the Open Division. Everyone gets thrown in there and it is tough to compete against athletes with visual or arm impairments, but two good legs. Some compete with a partner on a tandem bike. Tough competition for a CMT-affected athlete.

When we got back to Dallas, my sister-in-law gave me her pictures. One was of the swim start. She said they talked to me and I do not remember it. A CMT-affected athlete raced at Austin and said she talked to me. I have no memory of that conversation, either. She later joined Team CMT and plans to be at the National Championship next year.

Later, I saw a picture taken by the commercial photographer of me in my wetsuit, lying prone in the transition area. I look white as a sheet and am still surprised that I was allowed to race.

It is pretty scary I would get in the water the way I was affected. I think my training just kicked in once I hit the water. I so clearly remember the course and the place where I did the wrong turn last year. I remember the exit from the water. I remember talking myself through the swim using my swim mantra for face and breath, citing as I progressed on the course. 'Breathe"..."Stroke..."

I'm glad I came out of it okay and raced as well as I did. No excuses. Not a great performance, but I will just chalk it up to experience and things not to do again.

I met my family and returned to the hotel for a shower and the trip back to Dallas. I did not stay for the award ceremony. I was still angry and upset. Perhaps it was sour grapes, but I did not want my medal, which seemed a poor consolation for being shut out of the National Championship in the category in which I belonged, TRI 3. My time, even if I had a delayed start, would have put me in the top three. I might have earned a spot on Team U.S.A. and a trip to the World Championship in London. My time would have been good enough for second in the world last year. Despite my impaired state and possible late start, I was still competitive.

The race had ended, but my fight to gain acceptance as a CMT-affected athlete was just beginning. My advocates and I continue to work with the USAT.

No one has ever told me why I did not pass the assessment or how I don't meet an impairment of 15 percent. The more I corresponded with the manager of the USAT paratriathlon, the angrier I got. I also emailed the manager of the International Paratriathlon Union

She pointed her finger at the USAT and said it was up to the national body to certify athletes. The USAT said it was following ITU rules. The assessors had not been ITU-certified, so were they really following ITU rules or was the assessor I had making her own determination I did not belong?

Upset by the whole situation, I gave serious consideration to quitting triathlon competition all together. I had trained so hard and spent so much time, money, and energy to be ready. I was emotionally and physically exhausted. I wondered why I was putting myself through this experience.

Maybe it was time to do something else.

Chapter 96
When Do You Tell Someone?

If we are afraid to be different from the world, how do we expect to make a difference in the world?
—Reverend John Jenkins, past president of Notre Dame University

One day, I was with a couple of my friends and I mentioned my CMT symptoms. One of them said, "I don't' think you should tell anyone about your CMT." I think the friend meant not to tell someone when you are in a dating situation.

In truth, I was a bit offended by the advice, because telling someone about something like CMT is a highly personal decision. It isn't something anyone else can decide for you.

When do you tell someone you are dating you have a rare condition? When do you tell friends and co-workers about a condition that really isn't visible? I know from experience telling people about CMT can change the way they look at you.

In many ways, having CMT is not a big deal for me. My case is mild and I am doing really well. I am very fortunate compared to most people affected by CMT. I am active. In fact, I am really blessed to have run the Boston Marathon twice and competed at the National Paratriathlon Sprint Championship, even if it was in the open division. Many perfectly healthy athletes would love to have the opportunities I have had.

Sometimes, it can be difficult to tell others about my CMT because I do look perfectly fine. They have no idea of how tough it is to be an athlete and do some of the things I need to do to get through the day.

When I start to date someone, one of the first things I do is Google his name. I am sure he does the same. I've had lots of media coverage and am proud of my website. So hiding my CMT is not an option, at least not for long.

I would rather someone hear it from me instead of seeing my affliction on an Internet search. Besides I want to assure the guy how well I am doing. I have CMT, but it does not have me. I am still strong. I want to tell him about the work I am so excited and privileged to do.

I have told the last three men I have dated about my CMT early on in our relationship. If they are going to reject me because of my CMT, I would rather they do it early, before either one of us becomes emotionally involved. The first two said I was very brave. We did not date after they knew. The third will not even return my emails. At my age, it is tough to find men to date. They all seem to be looking for someone younger. Having CMT is not seen as an asset, either.

So I have been very open about having CMT. The funny thing is my family barely talks about CMT and I can't seem to shut up about it. In case you haven't noticed, I sometimes get a little obsessive when I get involved in something. When I am in, I'm all in.

I don't make a big deal about having CMT. Running in events like Boston makes it easy to bring up. Raising funds for CMT research makes it easy to tell others I have CMT as part of my campaign. It also helps I am not concerned about what people think of me. They are free to think whatever they want and I am not bothered by their opinions. If they think less of me because I have CMT, I feel that says more about them than about me. If they think I am a hero, well, I may not agree with that, but again, they are welcome to their opinions. I don't have the energy or desire to try and control what someone thinks about me. I do my best to be an open, honest, and considerate person. I know some people will not like me no matter what I do. I am not going to lose any sleep over it. I have enough problems sleeping the way it is.

Even non-athletes seem to know you need to qualify to run the Boston Marathon. Many ask me what my qualifying time was to get into the race. So when I talk about the race with them, it seems perfectly natural to tell them I am running in the Mobility Impaired Division and am raising money and awareness for charity. Many ask how I got involved with the charity. I tell them I have CMT and direct them to my website to learn more about the disease. It does not matter if they give; I have educated one more person about CMT.

It would seem hypocritical if I started a team to raise awareness and wasn't open to talking about my own CMT. I monitor several of the CMT-related groups on Facebook. One of discussions related a co-worker who thought she had MS. The group consensus was not to correct the co-worker. Many didn't think they should disclose their CMT to their co-workers. Many people with CMT never talk about it. They seem to be ashamed of the condition. How are we ever going to raise awareness unless we change this type of behavior?

Other times, I've seen members of Facebook groups talk about wearing their leg braces with shorts, then when asked about the braces, give out brochures about CMT. I hope someday it will be common to be so open about having CMT. It is something we were born with. We didn't do anything to get or deserve this disease. None of us have anything to be ashamed of.

I am passionate about raising awareness of CMT. No one should have to have a disease that causes you to slowly lose the use of your hands and legs and have someone stare at you when you tell them the name. It's like being victimized twice—first by the condition and then from lack of recognition and understanding. The least I can do is set a good example and be open about my own CMT. So yes, I will continue to be open about my CMT, even if it costs me dates and friends. It is a price I am willing to pay to make the public aware about CMT.

Chapter 97
The Finish Line

*Like the marathon, life can sometimes be difficult, challenging
and present obstacles, however if you believe in your dreams
and never give up, things will turn out for the best.*
—Meb Keflezighi , Olympic Marathon Silver medalist,
winner of New York Marathon

My experience in Austin left me emotionally and physically drained. For the second year, I had been discounted and dismissed as a physically challenged athlete. After the promises made to assess me based on the evidence we would present, I felt like Charlie Brown when Lucy pulls the football away at the last minute.

It is so difficult to know I can complete with the other athletes and be denied that chance. I had worked so hard to be ready, only to be disappointed yet again. I had to watch athletes with slower finishing times than mine claim spots on the U.S. team with the opportunity to go to the World Championships in London.

When I returned to Dallas with my family—angry, disappointed, and drained—I wondered why I should continue. I doubted whether I would ever make it through the classification process. It seemed no one in the United States with CMT was clearing the classification process, yet athletes with MS were. It all seemed so unfair. I was so frustrated because I felt as an athlete with CMT, I was not taken seriously.

I spent the week after Nationals in Dallas with my family. I always enjoy visiting my brother Tony's family. His wife Cindy and I are best friends. We shop and talk about her kids and our jobs.

The George W. Bush Presidential Library had just opened a few weeks earlier and Tony, Cindy, and I made a visit. I love history so I knew I would enjoy the opportunity.

One of the exhibits showed the visit to the White House by the Olympic and Paralympic teams. As I looked at the pictures, I knew I still had the desire to be on the U.S. team and maybe even go to Rio in 2016. I know it was a long shot but I still had the wish and the dream to pursue competition at the national level.

In 2016, I will be 58 years old. Not unheard of. A 71-year-old equestrian from Japan participated in the London Olympics in 2012. The oldest Olympian was a Swedish marksman who was 72 years, 280 days old. The current champ in my category is in her 40s. So just maybe I can stay competitive—now let's see if I can pass the classification process.

A few days after my revelation, I saw this quote on Facebook: *"You are not just waiting in vain. There is a purpose behind every delay."* Mandy Hale. Blogger turned hit author, Mandy Hale is affectionately known around the world as "The Single Woman" and is author of the *Single Woman's Sassy Survival Guide.*

I started my work raising awareness because I thought I had an interesting story to tell. In some ways, I've accomplished that, but there is so much yet to do.

I've learned to turn this effort over to God. Anything I accomplish will be on His timetable, not mine. Surrendering like that takes patience, something I never seem to have enough of.

Getting the USAT to recognize CMT is just part of the small fight those of us with CMT face every day. We are often told we look fine and others do not know about the struggle it can be to live with even a mild form of this condition.

So I will continue my fight. I don't know how to act any other way. I seem to have this need to right wrongs when I find them. The effort to be National Champion motivates me. As I continue my efforts, the rewards to be reaped include greater awareness and fundraising for CMT. So I will continue my training and work just as hard as I prepare for more appearances at national championship level events. I will run Boston again. I will continue to compete and raise awareness as long as my CMT allows me to do so.

I sense God still has a purpose and a plan for me and Team CMT. As of this writing, the Team has reached 137 members, all of whom have interesting stories to tell. Twenty-five of our athletes are affected by CMT. The members of this team will continue to prove the medical community wrong. Despite negative comments from some in the CMT community, we will continue our work.

Members of this team have done events that are a challenge for any athlete. Four of our team members have done Ironman Triathlons, and many run marathons and half-marathons. We are showing the world what someone with CMT can do.

When I found out I had CMT, I could not believe that 155,000 other Americans had this disease. That is as many as have MS. I could not believe I had never heard or CMT. I could not believe so many others were not aware of this disease. That did not seem right to me. I set to change that with my efforts and those of my Team CMT teammates.

On any given weekend, Team CMT members participate in events somewhere in the country. We have run high-profile events like the Boston Marathon, the Marine Corps Marathon, Ironman Florida, Dublin Marathon, Paratriathlon National Sprint Championship, and other events where thousands of spectators line the course.

Fredrick Douglas said "If there is no struggle, there is no progress." I have felt the struggle. I live the struggle. All of us with CMT have felt and lived the struggle. Now we work and hope for progress. We race always moving toward the finish.

I think about a line in one of my favorite Robert Frost poems. "But I have promises to keep and miles to go before I sleep."

In a marathon, the finish line seems far away. Sometimes it seems like treatments and a cure are far away as well. I know with hard work and commitment, we will get there. I know the members of Team CMT will be a large part of winning this battle.

Running a race like Boston or competing at the National Championship may seem like a little thing, but I know some how it is all connected to our fight for treatments and a cure. Just like the finish line, it can't come soon enough.

Acknowledgments

I f it takes a village to raise a child, then it takes a team, to keep a CMT-affected athlete healthy and able to compete.

It is quite a challenge to keep me competition ready and I have a great team of professionals, friends, and family members helping me. Thanks to my following team members:

Dr. Mark Drewicz of Chiropractic Associates has seen me through many running injuries and connected me to other in the triathlon and running community.

Dr. Robert Chetlin, PhD, is an exercise physiologist at the University of West Virginia Medical School. He helped me put together my training program for both Boston and the Paratriathlon Sprint Nationals in Austin in May. He has also been a tireless advocate for CMT-affected athletes before USA Triathlon.

Dr. Barczak is a former All American long-distance runner. He made the orthotics I have used in my running shoes for over 10 years. Because of the CMT, I am really prone to injury. For a long-distance runner, everything depends on your feet and a good set of orthotics are key to staying healthy.

The Sports Medicine Center of Froedert Hospital in Milwaukee is great. The folks there never ask you to stop running when you have an injury. Froedert is a teaching hospital, so I always seemed to have lots of residents and students peeking in as my case progressed. They have great physical therapists.

I also found a great physical therapist in Tom Brice at Athletico. He is a former Marquette Basketball player and athlete. He has actually heard of CMT and understands the challenges of being an athlete with this condition.

When I was accepted to compete at my first Paratriathlon event I knew I needed help. I then approached Florida USAT Level 1 Triathlon Coach Joy Von Werder. She is an Ironman finisher who has CMT. I don't have to explain anything to her. As an athlete, she knows what I go through. I email her every day and she has been with me through injuries and all the up and downs of being a CMT-affected athlete. She is my coach, advocate and fellow Team CMT member.

I so appreciate the advice and expertise of all these professionals. I hope they feel I am worthy of their time and attention.

There are countless others that have also helped me on my journey:

To Kira Henschel, my editor. Thank you for taking on this project and helping me to give a voice to those of us affected by CMT. You made the entire process including the editing fun and dealt with some unexpected drama around the book. Thank you for your support.

To Allison Moore, thank you for the sponsorship of the Hereditary Neuropathy Foundation. As a fellow athlete, you understand the importance of exercise to slow progression of CMT. Your vision and leadership in the CMT community is a model for many of us.

To author and friend Jon Helminiak. Your writing style has influenced my own. Thanks for the countless questions I asked about writing and publishing a book. Thank you for your encouragement as I worked to bring this book to life.

To dear friend Cheryl Monnat. You listened as I talked about starting this team and patiently looked at tee shirt designs for our uniforms. When many friends deserted me, you were steadfast in your friendship and support. You were my "first follower." You have been there for all the ups and downs of this journey and literally ran beside me in Boston. You have the rare ability to be excited about a friend's success. I know I can always count on you for friendship and support.

To my brother Tony and sister-in-law Cindy. Cindy, you got up at 4 a.m. to drive me to the triathlon in Denton, Texas, where I qualified for my first Paratriathlon National competition and Tony, you were there when I ran my first race as an HNF Team CMT member at the Allen Half-Marathon. Both of you have been with me at both Sprint Nationals in Austin. I have no family of my own, and you let me be a part of yours. Thank you for your love and support and being understanding when I go out for yet another run or bike ride when visiting my Texas family.

To my nephews, Brandon and Dan, you always make me laugh and remember not to take myself too seriously. I look forward to seeing what lies ahead for both of you.

To my beautiful and intelligent niece, Courtney. Your own courage in your fight with CMT inspire my own efforts. I run for you. I love you more than words can ever express.

To my brother Norbert and friend Ann. Thank you for being at the finish line at the Madison Marathon when I qualified for Boston. You knew my bad history with this race and were at the finish in your Team CMT tee shirts to bring me in. Your support means more than words can say.

Finally to Mom. You did not know about my CMT. I hope you would be proud of the person I have become and my work for CMT. You set the example of selfless sacrifice and love for others I strive every day to meet. I think of you and miss you every day.

Appendix

RECRUITING ATHLETES FOR TEAM CMT

Have you ever seen the big-name athletes in races and triathlons wearing their team uniforms? Wish you could be sponsored too or part of a team? You have a chance to join Team
CMT. Team CMT is now recruiting triathletes, runners,
duathletes, and fitness nuts to become members of Team CMT.

I am seeking team members to help me raise awareness of
Charcot Marie Tooth Disease, CMT. Worldwide, 2.6 million
people have this disease and most medical professionals of
never heard of it.

A few facts about CMT, the most common inherited
neuropathy, affecting 150,000 Americans. CMT is:

- Is a slowly progressive, causing deterioration of peripheral
  nerves that control sensory information and muscle
  function of the foot/lower leg and hand/forearm.

- Causes degeneration of the peroneal muscles (located on
  the front of the leg below the knee.

- Causes foot drop, walking gait problems, high arches,
  hammer toes, problems with balance, and problems with
  hand function, loss of normal reflexes and curvature of
  the spine.

- There is no effective treatment, although physical therapy
  and moderate activity are beneficial.

- It can in rare instances cause severe disability.

- CMT affects all genders and races.

If one parent has CMT, there is a 50 percent chance of getting the disease. The gene that causes CMT has been identified.

Please visit my website (http://www.run4cmt.com/) to raise funds for research and raise awareness. The main function of the Team CMT is to raise awareness. When you join Team CMT, you will receive a high-quality Eastbay running singlet with the Team CMT logo. We only ask you wear the singlet when competing, and then send a picture. Pictures will be posted on the Run 4 CMT Facebook page.

Take a moment to visit the website at http://www.run4cmt.com/ to learn about this effort. Select the Team CMT tab to see the singlet and join the effort. Our goal is a world without CMT. We are so close to a cure. Please help us get closer. Visibility means awareness. Awareness will be better diagnoses by the medical community and more funds for research.

CMT-AFFECTED ATHLETE

This summary shows the ways I am affected as an athlete in each of the triathlon disciplines. Most people with CMT would find being an athlete difficult, if not impossible. CMT symptoms can vary in severity, but the list below would be fairly typical for any athlete with CMT.

General

Symptoms can vary in type and severity among athletes; here are some general affects from my CMT:

- Swallowing issues that can cause me to aspirate fluids when drinking during workouts and competition. Any water in throat during the swim causes throat spasms.

- Muscle wasting is a characteristic of this disease. I have virtually no muscle at the wrists and ankles and diminished muscle mass in my arms.

- Incontinence caused by nerve damage. I have to wear pads when I run the fluid flow is so high.

- Balance issues, falls and ankle turning. Falls can happen unexpectedly and at any time.

- Fatigue. It takes twice as much energy for a CMT-affected athlete to do anything physical. It takes a nerve impulse twice as long to travel my extremities than a normal athlete. This can be measured with a nerve conduction test.
  So I expend more energy during workouts and competition. I start every race tired and feel like it will be a challenge to finish. I train longer and harder (usually twice the distance) to make up for this.

- Decreased sensation and feeling in hands, forearms and lower legs. This makes it hard to change technique and improve form since the sensory feedback is compromised. It takes longer to learn anything physical since it takes longer to build muscle memory. This can be measured with pin-prick tests and checking reflexes.

- Difficulty sleeping and staying asleep. Sleep disturbances are common with CMT patients. My body does not always get the rest it needs to recover from workouts.

- Increased risk of injury due to bio-mechanical issues (fractures and tendonitis are common).

- Difficulty regulating temperature so hands and feet are chronically cold. This also means the body has a hard time compensating for very hot temperatures. My body does not sweat as much so cooling is a problem in hotter temperatures.

- Loss of some dexterity in hands, making some tasks difficult such as buckling my helmet, applying race stickers, removing my wetsuit, tying shoes and changing shoes during transition, and so on.

- Muscle wasting can be seen at the wrists and ankles. Both my wrists and ankles have little mass. I can put my fingers around my wrists.

- My foot drop causes permanent muscle strain on the lateral sides of both ankles. I have developed a cyst on the right ankle due to the constant strain. There is pain when doing any of the triathlon activities.

Swim

- The swim kick is affected by lack of ankle flexibility. I do not get the full use of my leg muscles. My ankle flex on the right side is most affected; it is ½ of what it should be.

- I do not have good sensation in feet and hands, so body position can be off and I would not know. I was told recently I was spreading my fingers during my swim stoke. I had no idea due to the lack of sensation in my hands.

- It takes longer to improve technique and build muscle memory due to slow nerve conduction.

- Need to use a wetsuit since I get cold easily due to poor regulation of body temperature.

- Some difficulty with wet suit removal due to loss of strength in hands.

- Tripping at the start of the swim leg. Beaches are very uneven ground and the risk of a fall is higher for me than other athletes.

Bike

- I cannot flex my ankle to get a good pedal stroke when clipped into pedals.

- I cannot currently use aero bars due to balance issues.

- I have had several falls this season when biking. I recently switched to clip less pedals and cannot always un-clip my feet fast enough to prevent a fall. It takes me longer to develop muscle memory to make this second nature.

- Loss of feeling and sensation makes adjusting to road conditions and bike handling a challenge.

Run

- I cannot run every day due to the biomechanical issues (very tight hamstrings, Achilles tendon, high arches and hammertoes). If I run every day, I get injured. I got stress fracture training for my first marathon.

- The tightness in my lower legs means I cannot flex my foot enough to run with a proper gait. My leg swings from my hip to clear my foot drop. This means I do not get the power needed out of my legs. This means good running form is difficult. A good forward lean is difficult due to poor ankle flexibility.

- I get blisters from the twist in my stride, my feet burn when I run.

- The foot drop I have causes foot to drag, slowing me down. Also causes falls since I do not always clear obstacles like raised sidewalks or curbs.

- My biomechanics also are currently causing problems with my ankles. The ankle instability I have from lack of foot and leg flex are straining my ankles. I have developed a cyst in the right ankle and muscle pain in the left ankle.

- Last year, I wore my running orthotics on the wrong feet causing an injury. I could not tell since I have diminished sensation in my feet.

- Drastically decreasing times. I compare myself to a friend the same age. I train more. She runs a 10K in 51 minutes; I do it in right around 61 minutes. Our times when we started running together 20 years ago were almost identical.

- I had a bike accident 14 years ago. My running times dropped from 7:30 to 10:00 minutes. This happens when a CMT-affected athlete has an accident. My drop was immediate. It may be due to the 3 week layoff I had for surgery. I was once competitive in my age group. No longer due to this accident.

- During long runs my legs have significant pain. This is due to nerve damage.

- After a long run I will have difficulty sleeping because my legs are restless (jumpy, like being shocked) and my whole body feels like it is burning. All due to nerve damage.

An Open Letter to the CMT Community from Dr. Robert Chetlin

Research Update on CMT and Exercise

CMT Athletes, CMT Patients, CMT Families, and the CMT Community:

My name is Robert Chetlin. I am an associate professor in the Department of Human Performance and Applied Exercise Science in the West Virginia University School of Medicine. I also hold an appointment in the Department of Neurology at the same institution. For approximately the past 15 years, I have dedicated a significant portion of my time to study the effects of exercise in persons with CMT. Although you do not know me, I have been a supporter and member of Team CMT since its very beginning.

Many of you personally appreciate the benefits of exercise and provide testimonial that regular exercise helps maintain your strength, your endurance, your ability to carry out daily activities, and your quality of life.

Some studies we have done provide clear evidence that the muscle of some CMT patients beneficially responds to an exercise stimulus by increasing muscle size (called hypertrophy) and activating some of the proteins known to control muscle growth.

In CMT patients capable of exercise participation, regular exercise and activity reduces the risk of disease associated with a sedentary lifestyle, including Type 2 diabetes and heart disease.

In fact, many governmental and non-governmental agencies, namely the United States Department of Health and Human Services, the Office of the United States Surgeon General, the American Medical Association, and the American College of Sports Medicine, all agree that children and adults with chronic disease and disability, whom are capable, should engage in regular forms of exercise and activity. By definition, this would include a very large segment of the CMT patient population.

Despite the official position statements of these multiple nationally and internationally recognized and respected organizations, very few studies (less than two dozen), historically, have examined the effects of exercise in patients with various forms of CMT. As many of you are likely aware, the vast majority of CMT research has, up to this point, focused on discovery; that is, finding out about new types and subtypes of CMT and creating animal models of CMT. Though this type of science, called basic science, is valid and intriguing, CMT patients express little enthusiasm for these types of studies, because it is difficult to see the direct utility and benefit to patients themselves.

When patients I work with ask me how basic science will improve their daily lives, I am literally at a loss for words to provide an adequate explanation. It has been my experience that there exists a very palpable frustration amongst CMT patients today that the scientific community is so enamored with discovery that direct physical (non-surgical) treatment for patients has been relegated to a lower tier of importance. Other (non-physical) interventions have been attempted, namely drugs and nutritional supplements, but these have all failed to demonstrate long-term treatment effectiveness.

A thorough review of the scientific and clinical literature indicates that no drug or nutritional supplement, administered alone or in combination, has effectively treated or cured any degenerative and/or progressive neuromuscular disease or disorder, including CMT—perhaps the most complex and enigmatic neuromuscular disorder known to medical science.

So why haven't more studies been done to determine precisely how, and for whom, exercise may ultimately benefit CMT patients?

Quite simply, money; comparatively speaking, virtually all public and private funding has been devoted to the basic science of CMT. The result has been fewer physical interventional studies (including exercise), and the generation of smaller amounts of evidence to support regular exercise for capable CMT patients. In addition to defensive medicine, this "lack of evidence" is often cited, anecdotally, as to why many medical professionals advise against regular exercise and activity participation for their CMT patients.

Are there any circumstances or developments that promote a greater emphasis on studies that directly and comprehensively examine the effects of exercise on CMT disease?

Thankfully, that answer is "yes"! This is one of the reasons I have offered to write this narrative: to inform you about some exciting work and promising research on exercise and CMT.

A consortium of basic and clinical scientists has been formed between the National Institute for Occupational Safety and Health (NIOSH), the Max Planck Institute for Experimental Medicine (Gottingen, Germany), and the West Virginia University School of Medicine.

We propose to initially utilize experimental animals genetically modified to have CMT1a (the most common form of CMT), developed at the Max Planck Institute, by exposing them to a very controlled resistance-type exercise program on a machine called a dynamometer, developed at NIOSH. Upon completion of this validated animal exercise protocol, we will examine changes in the proteins, genes, and biochemicals associated with the nerves and muscles of the trained animals, as well as their strength and performance, and compare such change to non-exercising CMT control animals. We will be able to determine the precise effects of exercise from the genetic level to the performance level.

This research model will also allow us to: go back and better refine the exercise program; test animals with other forms of CMT (such as CMT2), and; include drugs or gene therapies with exercise, or both, to determine if the combination of drugs/gene therapies and exercise is more effective than any of these treatments administered alone. Ultimately, this body of evidence will be used to formulate an intervention strategy to be tested in human patients with CMT during Phase II of our research. Phase II will include studying a wide range of the CMT population: from those CMT patients wanting to increase their functional ability and improve the quality of their lives; to CMT athletes training to improve competitive performance, with or without a sport version of the Helios bracing system.

The collaborative, seminal (foundational) research just described is being made possible by the generous support of the Hereditary Neuropathy Foundation (HNF) and Team CMT, a group of CMT athletes and exercise enthusiasts, who, through athletic competition, raise the funds needed to drive this translational project.

Now, what can be done to support this novel research?

Everybody affiliated with the CMT community can help. If you are an athlete or exercise enthusiast with CMT, join Team CMT and fundraise; the money you raise through athletic competition will go directly toward the described exercise research. If you are a patient with CMT, have a loved one with CMT, or are otherwise involved in the CMT community, join HNF and donate whatever you can; indicate that your donation go directly to support CMT exercise research.

Lastly, here is my pledge to you: I will make myself personally available to answer whatever questions you may have regarding the information provided and what the future of CMT exercise research may hold. Most scientists wouldn't think of doing this, but changing the direction of CMT research is so profoundly important, I am willing to talk to you directly about our hopes and aspirations. I would also be happy to pass along any questions you may have for our collaborators at NIOSH or the Max Planck Institute for Experimental Medicine. Feel free to e-mail me at: rchetlin@hsc.wvu.edu.

Thank you for taking the time to read this.

Most sincerely,

Robert D. Chetlin, PhD, CSCS, CHFS
Associate Professor
Department of Human Performance and Applied Exercise Science
Department of Neurology
West Virginia University School of Medicine
PO Box 9139
Morgantown, WV 26506-9139

Team CMT in the news

Following are links to sound bites of Team CMT members discussing their experiences as runners with CMT:

CMT's effect on running
> http://www.youtube.com/watch?v=ngoMDCYVx-g&feature=youtu.be

Hereditary Neuropathy Foundation: Team CMT Leader to Run Boston
> http://www.help4cmt.com/articles/?id=110&pn=team-cmt-leader-to-run-boston-marathon

M Magazine: Boston Qualifier Running for a Cause

Media Milwaukee: Runner Transcends Challenges
> http://www4.uwm.edu/mediamilwaukee/culture/runner.cfm

NOW: BayView woman with neurological challenge trains for dream marathon, February 23, 2012
> http://www.bayviewnow.com/userstoriessubmitted/140141793.html

Peninsula Pulse: When Every Step is a Challenge
> http://www.ppulse.com/Articles-c-2011-05-03-97495.114136-When-Every-Step-Is-A-Challenge.html

Runner's Sole: Sharing Stories of Inspiration
> http://runnerssole.co.uk/christine-wodke.html

Silent Sports Magazine: When Every Step is a Challenge
> http://www2.silentsports.net/content/running/stories/cmt-sufferer-wodke-11-2011.php

Silent Sports Magazine: A 2013 Runner's Thoughts on the
Boston Marathon
http://www.silentsports.net/running/a-2013-boston-marathoners-
thoughts-jcpg-325466-209778341.html

TeamCMT educates, informs
http://www.youtube.com/watch?
v=eJY6YZc8Mg0&feature=youtu.be

TriDigest: Triathletes Unite to Raise Awareness of Charcot-
Marie-Tooth
Tri Digest
http://tridigest.com/triathletes-unite-to-raise-awareness-of-charcot
-marie-tooth

Whitefish Bay Patch: Friends Unite to Run Toward a Cure
http://whitefishbay.patch.com/articles/friends-reunite-to-run-
toward-a-cure

WTMJ News (Milwaukee) Interview with Trenni Kusinerek
http://www.620wtmj.com/blogs/trennikusnierek/141808943.html

CMT Resources

Hereditary Neuropathy Foundation
www.hnf-cure.org

National CMT Resource Center
http://www.help4cmt.com/

MDA- Muscular Dystrophy Association
http://mda.org/

Neuropathy Now Magazine, American Academy of Neurology
http://patients.aan.com/go/neurologynow

Team CMT
www.run4cmt.com
Blog: http://run4cmt.blogspot.com/
Email: Run4cmt@yahoo.com
Facebook: Run4CMT
Twitter: Run4CMT
YouTube Channel: www.youtube.com/run4cmt

CMT UK
http://www.cmt.org.uk/

Prescription Drugs and CMT

National CMT Resource Center
http://help4cmt.com/articles/?id=138&pn=neurotoxic-drugs-and-charcot-marie-tooth-disease

National Institute of Health
http://www.ninds.nih.gov/disorders/charcot_marie_tooth/charcot-marie-tooth_fs.pdf

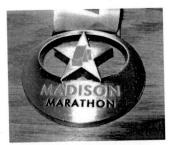

Madison finisher medal

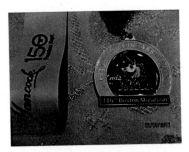

2012 Boston finisher medal

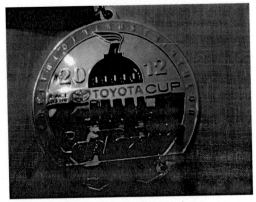

National Championship medal

About the Author

C hristine Wodke is the founder and manager of Team CMT, a group of 123 athletes from 27 states working to raise awareness of Charcot-Marie-Tooth Disorder, or CMT. The mission of Team CMT is to raise awareness about CMT and raise funds for research. In addition, Chris is a chemical engineer and JOB DESCRIPTION

A Milwaukee native who was diagnosed in 2010 with CMT, Wodke puts many Baby Boomer women to shame with her physical fitness, and maintains it all while fighting side-effects of CMT. These include structural and muscular challenges with bouts of tripping, burning sensations in her feet, and atrophy.

Wodke has been a competitive runner for over twenty years and took on the challenge of doing triathlons three years ago. She has completed eight marathons and countless half-marathons.

She is a two-time participant of the Boston Marathon. She was running the Boston Marathon in 2013 when the blasts occurred.

Accomplishments / RACE Resume

- Boston Marathon, April 15, 2011, 2nd Mobility Impaired Division, finish time 5 hr 27 minutes

- Boston Marathon, April 16, 2012, projected finish: 5 hr 15 min

- Cap Tex Tri, May 26, 2012
  1st Open Physically Challenged Division

- Paratriathlon National Sprint Championship, 1:39:43

- Cap Tex Tri, May 27, 2013
  2nd Open Physically Challenged Division
  Paratriathlon National Sprint Championship
  750 m swim, 20 K bike, 5K run
  1 hr 46 minute

- Pleasant Prairie Triathlon, June 23, 2013
  1st Paratriathlon Ambulatory Division Sprint
  Triathlon, 750 m swim, 20 K bike, 5 K run, 1:43:47

- Pewaukee Lake Triathlon, July 14, 2013
  1st Paratriathlon Division, 500 m swim, 14.8 mile
  bike, 5 K run, 1:41:33

- Midwest Regional Paratriathlon Championship,
  First Paratriathlon Division, July 21, 2013, Omaha,
  Nebraska, 750 m swim, 20K bike, 5K run, 1st
  Place Female, 1:41:08

- USAT Age Group National Championship,
  August 11, 2013, Milwaukee, Wisconsin
  750 m Swim, 20K bike, 5K run
  1 hr 41:07, 32 out of 44 women

- Chicago Triathlon—Paratriathlon Mid-east
  Regional Championship, August 25, 2013
  750 m Swim, 14 mile bike, 5K run,
  1st place Female TRI 3, 1 hr 51:45

- Tri Rock Sprint Triathlon Lake Geneva, September
  14, 2013, 500 Meter Swim, 14.8 mile bike, 5K run,
  1st place Female Paratriathete, 1 hr 49:05

Although she tires easily from effects of CMT, you'll seldom
hear her complain or use it as an excuse.

CPSIA information can be obtained
at www.ICGtesting.com
Printed in the USA
FFOW04n2050201213
2742FF